THE CROHN'S DIARIES

A BOOK OF RESILIENCE

Meagan Davey

For my grandfather Kevin,
a much-loved fellow chronic illness warrior.
One of the strongest people I know…

CONTENTS

Author's notes...i

   The little superscript numbers......................................i

   On products...i

Why I decided to write this book iii

INTRODUCTIONS...1

   So, what is Crohn's disease anyway?......................1

   My story...3

PART ONE 11

   Post-operative stoma management......................13

   Troubleshooting tips that worked for me post-stoma
   surgery 15

   Management of minor stoma blockages..............16

   The art of balancing ileostomy output and maintaining
   adequate hydration...18

   My top tips for stoma management 21

   Bonus Bite!...22

  Meagan's Stoma-friendly Bircher 23

  Meagan's Stoma-friendly Chia Porridge 25

PART TWO...27

So, what is psoriasis?...29

How psoriasis & skin issues have affected my life 30

Managing chronic splits in my perianal skin.....................32

Psoriasis on my knuckles 33

Peristomal (the skin around the stoma) psoriasis.................34

My usual daily routine since the psoriasis has healed...........36

Bonus Bite!...37

Psoriasis of the navel..38

Periorificial dermatitis..40

PART THREE..45

Management of various perianal problems...........................47

Anal spasms: treat the spasm, treat the pain 48

Anal discharge: baby wipes 49

Discharge leakage prevention: makeup pads 49

Decreasing pain caused by anal wounds: salt baths 49

Bonus Bite!...50

Pubic pustules 51

PART FOUR..53

PART FIVE 61

Tips on how to assert yourself more...................................64

The 'Take-Aways'..65

PART SIX...67

Helpful Tips 71

SO HERE WE ARE… 73

SHARING THEIR STORIES 77

    INTERVIEW WITH A FELLOW CROHN'S
    FIGHTER 77

    Melissa Lord (@gutlessandwonderful) 79

MEAGAN'S SURVIVAL SHOPPING LIST 87

    Bonus Bite! 89

REFERENCES 91

GLOSSARY 95

AUTHOR'S NOTES

The little superscript numbers

There are quite a few medical terms thrown around in this book e.g. gastroenterologist[1]. If the definition is too large, or the term needs further explanation, I have done so in the Glossary at the very back of the book. Match the little number next to the term to the corresponding number in the Glossary.

On products

I will be naming the products I use in my self-care routines as I personally believe in them and have found them to be very helpful in managing my conditions over the years. I also feel good using these products because the majority, though not all of them, are made of natural ingredients, and contain minimum preservatives.

I am constantly reviewing the products I use and exploring and trialling new ones to achieve the best balance between all-natural ingredients and the results I need for my body.

I am not endorsing these products for financial gain or to push a sale. I am simply sharing what has worked and continues to work for me. Finding the right products for you is very important and often involves a fair bit of trial and error. If you find a particular product that works for you personally, by all means use it!

You can find my handy Meagan's Survival Shopping List of the products I mention at the back of the book with links to information and online suppliers.

WHY I DECIDED TO WRITE THIS BOOK

I never had any intentions of writing a book – it just happened one day. I was sharing some psoriasis management advice with another Crohn's sufferer who was struggling with her skin issues at the time and had put the call for help out on Instagram. After giving her my advice based on my own experience and what helped for me, I realised that I actually have a wealth of knowledge on managing this illness and it would be a shame (and a waste) not to pass my knowledge on to those in need.

After reading various information booklets and resources on Crohn's over the years, I realised that many only talk about the text book symptoms of the disease (which I did not suffer from) and the standard medical treatments recommended by the experts. They barely, *if at all*, touch on the secondary conditions, issues and complications that can develop as a result of having Crohn's.

These include, but are not limited to:

Physical issues involving the surgical site such as hernias and infection, the skin (i.e. psoriasis), the eyes, the joints, the liver, the kidneys;

Mental health issues such as anxiety and depression (guilty!) due to the strain of dealing with the condition day in and day out;

Financial issues and loss of income, i.e. having no sick leave remaining or the sadly real possibility of losing a job due to being unwell for periods of time and being unable to work.

So, I just started writing bullet points listing the products I use and detailing techniques I've developed over the years regarding managing my psoriasis and my stoma bag. All of a sudden, I began typing it up on my laptop and it naturally evolved from there.

I thought, hang on a minute – I've written this much already, why not just make it into an e-book?! After telling my life coach what I had done and what I was planning to do, she recommended an editor to me who fortunately agreed to come along on this journey.

Then one day I was having a meeting with my editor nearer to publishing, and we suddenly decided it needed pictures throughout and then ideas started firing regarding cover art concepts etc. My editor recommended a very skilled artist friend of his who happily agreed to jump on board and breathe life into my concepts for the cover art as well as the original drawings you will find within.

Now, here we are. I'm still in awe of how just a handful of bullet points had snowballed with great momentum into a resource that will hopefully really assist people suffering from Crohn's disease and the associated problems!

This book's purpose is threefold…

For the Crohnies

First and foremost, this book is dedicated to all of you Crohn's warriors.

For those of you with Crohn's and the related issues I speak about, think of this book as a trouble-shooting manual or guide that you can refer to as you please. Take what resonates and leave the rest. I truly hope this honest (and at times humorous) resource is a breath of fresh air for those who truly understand – those of you, just like me, who are battling day to day.

For the newly diagnosed, I understand the topics I write about may be too confronting right now, as it is perhaps unchartered territory for you. If this is the case, then only read this if and when you are called to. The intention of this book is not to scare you, it's to help prepare and empower you in the face of this disease. The subjects I speak about may or may not touch you personally during your lifetime, but knowledge really is your friend and developing a close relationship with yourself is key. This book highlights and celebrates the uniqueness of every single individual under the Crohn's umbrella and for this reason - what works for one will not work for all so start tuning in and learn to trust yourselves.

For the Crohn's tribe as a whole - of everything I have written about - three of the biggest messages I want to convey to you all are:

You are NOT your disease.

Your body is doing the BEST it can.

I see a lot of Crohn's related memes on social media demonising our bodies and I've realised that it doesn't sit well with me. Please don't hate on your body! It is doing the best it can and will continue to do so tirelessly every day until the day that you leave this earth.
Our bodies are actually pretty amazing.

You are all STRONGER than you know.

Be kind to, and proud of, yourselves!

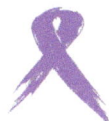

For those with Crohnies close to their hearts

I also dedicate this book to those of you who are always there for us Crohn's Warriors—the silent legends in the background (our friends, our families, our significant others). Thank you for believing we were sick when no one else would. Thank you for advocating for us when we are too sick and exhausted to do it ourselves. Thank you for continuously dishing out the unconditional love and support that we all need so much on our individual journeys. Thank you for continuing to be there for us even when we, in the grips of our illness, lash out and unfairly take it out on you. Thank you for just being you, often without the acknowledgement you deserve. Crohn's doesn't just affect us as individuals, it affects everyone close to us. They feel what we feel. If I haven't said it enough in the past – I am grateful for every single one of you legends in my own support circle!

For the Crohn's-curious

On my own Crohn's journey, I have experienced my fair share of unintentionally insensitive and unhelpful comments such as: "but you look so well", "are you sick *again*?", "should you be eating that?", "you are so lucky you can eat whatever you want and stay so skinny", "you shouldn't be consuming gluten or dairy", "how can you be tired, you sleep your life away", "but you're too young to be experiencing all these health problems", etc.

For me, this book acts as a window into the day-to-day life of a chronic disease warrior. It's an honest snapshot of the life of a Crohnie, where we all experience daily challenges, even those of us who are in remission right now. Challenges – whether they be in the form of: chronic fatigue, digestive issues, chronic pain, suffering an active flare-up, endless toilet trips, malaise, dehydration, surgical complications, stoma bag accidents, medication complications, mental health struggles, financial struggles, self-esteem and body image struggles, dating and relationship struggles, and so on and so forth.

It takes so much work to present 'normally' in society. I often think of chronic disease as a full-time job. I hope in writing this book I have been able to spread awareness throughout the non-Crohn's population in a gentle and non-judgemental way. I think it's also an important reminder for the global human community, Crohn's and non-Crohn's sufferers alike, that none of us truly know what individuals struggle with behind closed doors. So, lastly, I'd like to thank you as a non-Crohn's member of society for expressing your curiosity and wanting to learn about Crohn's disease from the perspective of the sufferer.

* * *

In writing this, I really want to spotlight the unique diversity of every individual, even when we are all standing beneath the global Crohn's umbrella. I cannot stress enough how incredibly important, and necessary, it is that you really get to know, and become in tune with, your own body; to take responsibility for your own health and health management *because you are the only one who knows how* you feel and how your body works. We all need to learn how to self-advocate and become assertive if we want to feel listened to and gain access to the best quality of life possible for ourselves (including mentally and emotionally).

In no way am I suggesting that you shouldn't follow medical advice in treating Crohn's because that is completely untrue. They are amazing at treating the big issues with medications and surgeries, which I have experienced my fair share of. I owe a lot to, and am grateful for, my gastroenterologist[1], my colorectal surgeon[2], my inflammatory bowel nurses and my stoma[3] nurses[4] and I have a great deal of respect for, not only their knowledge and expertise, but for, them as individuals.

I have learned a lot from them throughout the years. I am, however, trying to put across the fact that those of us with chronic illnesses do eventually become our own experts due to living with a multitude of issues every day and learning what works for us. We often work out how to manage a lot of the side issues related to the disease and/or our stomas for, and by, ourselves. All the day-to-day things that the experts don't really understand or know how to deal with.

So, I repeat - we, as individuals, have a key role to play and it is so important that we listen to our guts and follow our intuition regarding our own health. We know our own bodies better than anyone else!

In this resource I will share my story and my personal experience of what I have found that works for me in managing my stoma, my skin and pelvic issues, and my anxiety. Again, this doesn't mean that what works for me will work for you. I am not a doctor, but I hope I may give you some insight, ideas and helpful tips on what you can try for yourself and possibly, if they help, incorporate into your own health management plan.

If you decide to try one of my approaches but feel unsure, by all means, consult your medical professional to ensure it is safe to incorporate in combination with your current treatment.

If this resource helps just one person, I will be happy that I decided to pass on the information that I have been given and that I have myself learned so far.

INTRODUCTIONS

So, what is Crohn's disease anyway?

Inflammatory bowel disease (IBD), is an umbrella term that includes both Crohn's Disease and Ulcerative colitis. While both Crohn's and Ulcerative colitis are grouped together, there are quite significant differences between the two conditions.

Crohn's is an inflammatory autoimmune disease[5] that predominantly affects the G.I. (gastrointestinal) tract and can affect all layers of the intestinal wall (i.e. not just the lining), from mouth to anus. Inflammation can occur in the form of ulceration[6] or stricture[7] (narrowing) anywhere along the G.I. tract. IBD is often confused with Irritable Bowel Syndrome (IBS), Crohn's is not an IBS - they are different afflictions.

Like many chronic conditions, Crohn's disease is so much more multi-faceted than just being limited to the physical symptoms. Also, it is key to understand that every individual presents differently depending on where the Crohn's manifests in the GI tract and because of many other variables. Subsequently, it is essential that treatment, and even self-management, needs to be individualised for every person because one size certainly does not fit all!

If the condition becomes unresponsive to medical treatments (such as corticosteroids[8], immunomodulators[9] or biologics[10]), often the next step is surgery, sometimes multiple procedures, to remove the diseased portion of tract. As Crohn's is incurable, surgery does not guarantee there will not be a re-emergence of the condition.

This often results in a chronic cycle of recurring symptoms and active disease, generally referred to as a 'flare up'.

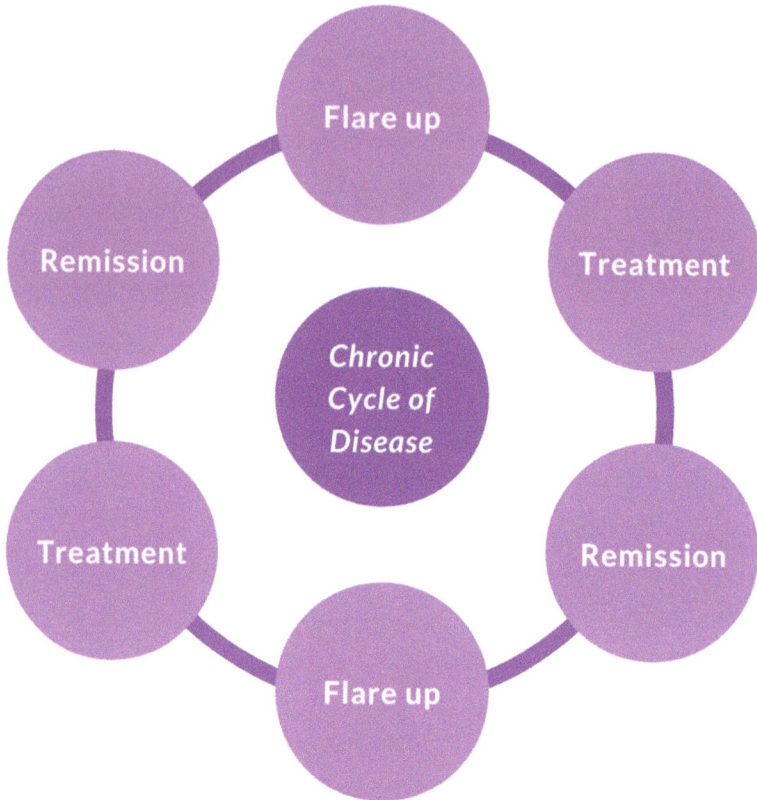

Flare up

Treatment

Remission

Chronic Cycle of Disease

Treatment

Remission

Flare up

It also unfortunately doesn't just affect the bowel. Crohn's is often associated with psoriasis and other skin conditions; it can inflame the joints (potentially causing arthritis); cause issues with the eyes and organs such as the liver and kidneys; cause mouth ulcers, perianal[11] fissuring[12] and ulceration; fistulas[13], bowel obstructions and perforations[14]; compromise the immune system; and the list goes on. (NIDDK)

My story

As a chronic disease sufferer, my story is quite extensive, and as such, I have excluded some of the events and issues I have experienced along the way.

Including, the multiple disease flares, all of my many procedural complications, the hellish recovery from my 2013 surgery, the total depletion of my sick leave on numerous occasions, the inability to work at different periods, and having to apply for income protection and live off 75% of my base wage a number of times. Not to mention the separation of my parents and death of my father thrown in as well.

Why? Because, frankly, I would be writing about it forever. I have chosen, instead, to focus on the significant points I have encountered along the path that has brought me to this moment, typing out my story with hope in my heart that it will resonate with anyone out there also struggling through their own chronic disease challenges.

In 2007, at the age of 20, I was diagnosed with Crohn's Disease - predominantly of the terminal ileum[15] and perianal area, in, and around, my anus, with a few patches in the sigmoid colon[16]. However, looking back, I realise how unwell I had been for many years before that.

From the age of 12, symptoms of lethargy, light-headedness, chronically elevated liver enzymes[17], constipation, abdominal pain, chronic anal fissuring and inflammation had begun to appear. Despite these symptoms, I was otherwise healthy and active, playing a fair amount of sport throughout my early years including swimming and netball.

Prior to diagnosis I had started to become paranoid and anxious that I had a terminal illness because of the symptoms I was constantly experiencing. So, Mum took me to see a number of different gastroenterologists whose only action was an endless chain of blood tests. They all believed an endoscopy and colonoscopy (camera down the food pipe and into the bowel) was too invasive for a child of my age.

At that time neither my mum, nor I, had even heard of Crohn's Disease, so we just followed the specialist's advice.

Then, in 2006, I developed a painful fissure, and subsequent swelling, in my bottom and this time it never healed. I was referred to a colorectal surgeon, whom I still see to this day (although much less frequently) and was placed on a course of antibiotics. The antibiotics didn't heal the fissure, so the next step was a colonoscopy and endoscopy, ultimately revealing the bad news.

I remember the look of concern on my surgeon's face when he delivered the news; though I didn't really take the disease seriously at the start, because I, like most people, didn't know what Crohn's was or what terrible things it was capable of.

Funny but true story - I had begun working on a Crohn's presentation for my nursing training the very week I received my diagnosis!

Post diagnosis, my initial drug therapy was balsalazide (Colazide)[18] capsules. I did not notice a difference in symptoms with this medication, so I was then prescribed an immunomodulator called azathioprine (Imuran). It was not even a year later, in 2008, I experienced the first of many Crohn's flares (with symptoms including: erythema nodosum - red painful sores on my shins, severe vomiting, diarrhoea and abdominal pain) and was hospitalised. This was where I met my gastroenterologist, whom I continue to see now.

After 10 days in hospital, being loaded up on IV hydrocortisone and IV fluids, my medication was changed again, and I was discharged on prednisone and mercaptopurine tablets. I was also commenced on IV infliximab (Remicade) infusions. This was my first exposure to the joy of prednisone—I put on 10kg and developed a large appetite and an impressive 'moon-face'. A few rounds of infliximab later, Medicare informed me they would cease covering the drug costs because I was "no longer sick enough"!

My perianal disease worsened from then on, and by 2010, after an invasive investigation of the area under general anaesthetic, it was revealed that I had developed deep anal fissures, as well as an ulcer and large skin tags[19] around the anus. The pain of this was off the scale.

It hurt to sneeze, cough, bend over or get up, and I experienced constant faecal ooze from my bottom after every bowel movement. I was completely miserable and as my condition worsened, I was considered eligible to recommence the infliximab infusions—yeah thanks!

One week after restarting infliximab I developed myositis[20], severe muscle aches, which started as pain in my right shoulder, progressing to both arms, until I couldn't even lift my arms due to the weakness and pain. Off to the emergency department I went and was admitted straight away because my muscles had started to break down and there was a risk of developing rhabdomyolysis[21] which can cause severe kidney damage.

I was in hospital for five days while being pumped full of IV fluid to help my kidneys filter out the by-products of my damaged muscles. It was decided that I was to no longer continue with the infliximab in case it had caused this muscle issue. Instead, I was changed over to adalimumab (Humira) injections. Not for long though, as my blood results indicated the level of muscle damage was worsening so then the Humira was also ceased because it was thought to be playing a part.

As I was continuing to have muscle issues, and unable to take any of the big gun biologic medications to bring my flare under control, I was facing the real possibility of needing to have a bowel resection, meaning a portion of my bowel would be removed, and/or, a temporary loop ileostomy[22], constructed to rest my colon and perianal area to achieve "remission". The ileostomy meant I would have to use a Stoma bag[23] for the rest of my life.

When I first heard the mention of surgery, the doctor basically said something along the lines of, "You'll more than likely end up having surgery, most Crohn's patients do."

The delivery was so blunt and matter-of-fact, that I went into a state of shock. Once I had finished with the doctor that day I burst into tears in the corridor. I wasn't ready to take the reality of surgery on-board, and was so scared of what might happen, all the unknown possibilities.

At the age of 23, the thought of having to deal with "a bag" for the rest of my life just seemed too much. Why should I have to make this kind of life changing decision when I had no real idea about what was happening to me?

Around this time, I underwent a muscle biopsy of my right thigh to see what was causing the myositis and I saw a neurologist[24] after that for the results. The neurologist's opinion was that the infliximab had probably caused the original muscle issue and when I was swapped to the Humira the blood tests indicating muscle damage had merely trended up before ultimately decreasing and stabilising. They advised that I could retrial the Humira and recommence it if there were no further problems.

2011 came around, and despite being on long-term prednisone and Humira, the Crohn's in my colon and perianal area had worsened and I was in a lot of pain every day. Even though it had not been all that long since the Doctor had dropped the surgery bomb on me, I think back to how, by this stage, it was as if I had become a completely different person. I was almost begging them to do whatever it would take to get rid of my pain, even if it was with surgery.

So, it was then decided that I would undergo a temporary loop ileostomy construction to allow my faecal matter to be bypassed away from the diseased areas of my bowel in the hope of resting those areas and allowing the medications to gain control over the flare.

I had my surgery in August 2011 and during the procedure it was also discovered that I had endometriosis[25], no wonder I had been getting painful, heavy periods for years! (This is a whole other ongoing story).

After my surgery, further investigations into my muscle issues were made and a second muscle biopsy was taken from my thigh because the first test they had performed didn't look at the specific genetic makeup of the muscle. Results revealed that the reason I was having episodes of myositis was not due to my Crohn's medications but because I was/am in fact a symptomatic carrier of the Duchenne muscular dystrophy gene[26]. This means that if I had a son, I could pass the disease on to him and if I had a daughter, I could pass the carrier gene onto her and she could end up having a son with muscular dystrophy. This means In Vitro Fertilisation (IVF)[27] for me if I want to have children which, luckily, at this stage of my life, I don't.

Despite a short period of feeling well and not being in pain, by 2013 the combination of the Humira, prednisone and having the temporary ileostomy just wasn't effective in controlling my perianal disease. I was experiencing a lot of perianal skin breakdown and excruciating pain when passing mucus[28] from my bottom. Eventually, a large build-up of mucus was caught at my tailbone level because of my anus and rectum becoming so narrowed from disuse. The build-up caused intense pain in my tailbone and I could no longer lie on my back. The discharge had become dark, thick and smelled revolting from sitting in there for too long.

After a multitude of scopes, Magnetic Resonance Imaging (MRI's)[29], Computerised Axial Tomography (CT's)[30] and lengthy discussions with my gastroenterologist and colorectal surgeon, it was mutually agreed upon that more surgery was the only option to choose in preserving my quality of life. In December 2013, I underwent a laparoscopic pan proctocolectomy[31] (removal of large bowel, rectum and anus) with no modification to my stoma as it had been working well with no issues. My rectum, anus and internal anal sphincters[32] were removed, leaving only my external sphincters.

Let me tell you, as soon as I woke up after my surgery, I was sick as a dog. I literally woke up in the recovery room dry retching and feeling beyond terrible. The nausea and vomiting were partially caused by the IV pain relief; and partially due to the after effect of having a large amount of bowel removed. The pain-relief pump was taken down two days after the surgery because I just couldn't tolerate it, and besides, it wasn't actually helping reduce my pain.

I was bed-bound for the first week with the crippling combination of nausea, vomiting and constant pain. I was only allowed clear fluids[33] and lost at least 3 kilograms in 4 days. I preferred to sleep the days away instead of being awake and feeling what I was feeling. To this day, I would rather have pain over nausea any time!

Toward the end of that first week I developed a fever and began to feel really under par. They got the fever under control in hospital and despite telling staff that I didn't feel right and that I didn't think I was ready to go home yet; I was discharged home. The nurse in charge argued with me, stating that my observations were fine and that I didn't need to stay in hospital.

Low and behold, the very same evening I was discharged, I developed severe pain and spasms in my abdomen, sharp pains in both groins, diarrhoea bucketing from my stoma and another fever. I remember screaming out in pain and Mum calling the ambulance to take me back to hospital as I could not move off my bed.

In the emergency department, I was immediately placed on IV antibiotics, they got pain relief into me, and I had a scan of my abdomen and pelvis. The scan revealed that there was an infection developing in my pelvis from the surgery. I stayed in hospital while my surgical team was deciding what the best course of action would be. They didn't want to take me back into surgery so my stitches in my bottom wound were opened at my hospital bed with the idea that the infected discharge would drain by itself from my pelvis through the bottom and eventually heal up.

This approach didn't really go as planned.

The antibiotics I had received had killed off the bacterial growth causing the infection, however, from 2013-2015, I experienced chronic pelvic pain and a sensation of pressure as the collection of discharge would build up and my bottom would ooze a thick mucus-like substance from the sinus[34] (tunnel) where my rectum/anus was. It was uncomfortable, messy and embarrassing.

In an attempt to drain this collection and heal my pelvis, multiple drains were inserted, via the bottom wound causing multiple terrible complications. They also inserted one terribly painful drain (the CT guided trans-gluteal drainage approach[35]) that entered via my bottom cheek, was then fed through an open channel in my pelvis (via the sciatic foramen[36]) and inside my pelvic space to where the collection was sitting. This was performed while I WAS AWAKE! I will never forget the noises of the instruments used and the sensations I felt during that procedure.

Ultimately, these procedures proved unsuccessful. Although, at the time of each insertion, the pelvic pressure and pain would ease, once they were removed, the discharge built up again and pain would return.

I still experience episodes of pelvic pain and the mucus-like discharge draining from the now fully established sinus running from the original site of infection within my pelvis and exiting from the sinus in my bottom. I became so traumatised from, and sick of having, these procedures that I refused to have any more in 2015 and I have now just learned to accept it, manage it and live with it, knowing that I will never be 100%.

If I waited until I was 100%, I would never have achieved anything in my life. I would never have travelled overseas multiple times, I would never have dated anyone, and I certainly would never have had the quality of life I am experiencing right now! Sometimes the more we interfere with our bodies in an attempt to 'fix' them, the more long-term issues we continue to experience.

I'm happy to say that this is 'my normal' now and it's never stopped me from doing what I want to do. I've travelled around parts of Australia, to Fiji, India, Japan, Italy, Greece, Malta, and New

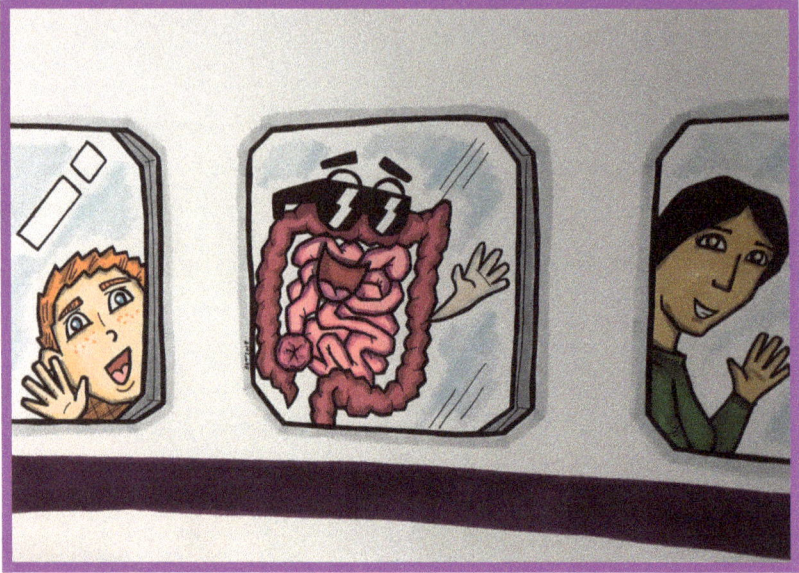

Zealand, and soon I will be off to Spain. A lot of these trips have been while I've been unwell, and with my pelvic drains in place! Can't keep a Crohnie down!

I thought, *if I don't travel now, when will I?*

PART ONE

STOMA ADVICE & TROUBLE SHOOTING

Post-operative stoma management

The process of recovery after having a stoma surgically created (in my case, having firstly a temporary loop ileostomy created in 2011,

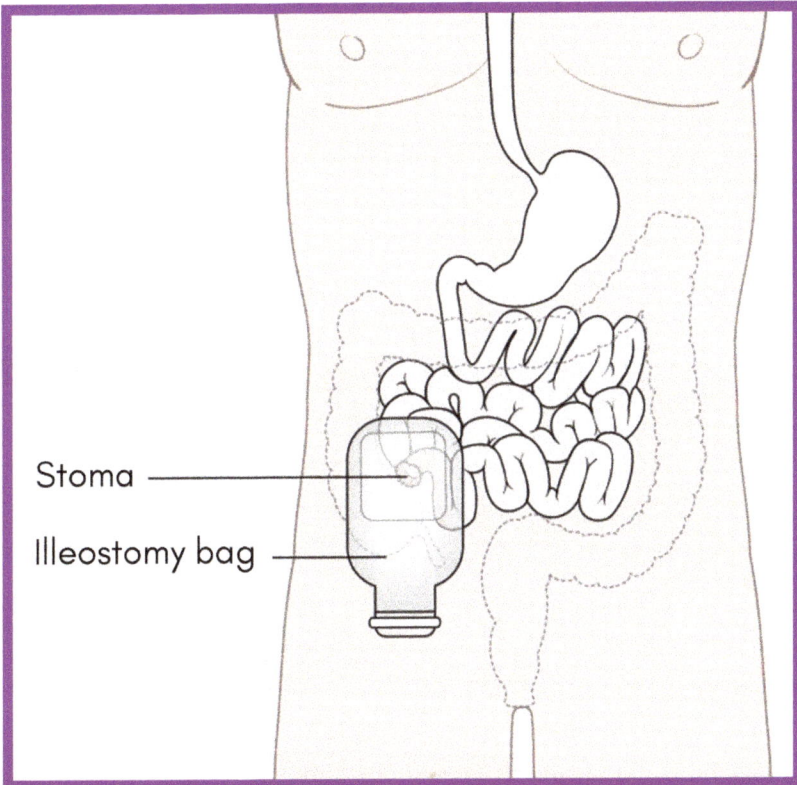

Stoma ——————

Illeostomy bag ——————

and then the ileostomy becoming permanent in 2013) requires a lot of tuning-in to your body and a lot of patience.

"Slow and steady wins the race", definitely applies here!

Let's consider exactly what your body has just been through. You've undergone a general anaesthetic and had pain medications administered, both during the surgery as well as post-op. Your abdominal wall and intestines have been cut open. The areas where the intestine have been cut are swollen and have been weakened as a result. You've been fasting for hours, possibly days, before surgery and you have been generally inactive since becoming sick and while in hospital.

All these factors are going to affect your bowel function for some time. Whether it be sluggish digestion, getting full really easily, feeling nauseated and/or actually vomiting, or, the bowel/stoma going on strike and not working at all.

It really makes sense why people are put onto a fluid diet first and then monitored before trialling more solid foods. It all takes time for the bowel to recover and it's not the sort of thing you want to try and rush through!

Sooo, let's explore my newbie's approach to recovery after my first surgery in 2011. I was up and walking around the day after my operation, in great spirits, and even made it down to the hospital cafeteria with my family. That evening, I proceeded to scoff down a large dinner and despite the fact I felt a bit too full to finish it, I ignored that feeling and forced down the last of the chicken breast, thinking nothing more of it.

Until…a couple of hours later, when I started feeling really bloated and nauseated. Then I started vomiting profusely and continued vomiting overnight. I was pumped full of anti-nausea medication (which I came to realise later was heightening my anxiety and inducing panic attacks) and IV fluids. I was in so much pain across my ribs and surgical sites from the strain of vomiting for hours. My high spirits quickly dissolved into misery and anxiety.

The next day I felt completely drained and depressed. My bowel was still sluggish and the combination of not chewing the chicken properly, not taking my time with it, and eating too much of it, had caused a slight blockage. If only I had tuned in and listened to my body when I was getting that 'full' signal and stopped eating there and then.

After that episode, I became quite scared to eat anything, I barely finished my meals while still in hospital. I would just try bites of things and thoroughly chewed it before I swallowed. Anything to avoid going through the hell of the previous day.

I gained valuable guidance from my stoma nurses and consciously started tuning into my body, letting it guide me during my recovery regarding things like; what and how much I ate, as well as what I did to avoid feeling sick after meals etc. Eventually I recovered really well and continued being careful with foods I ate until I felt comfortable and confident in knowing what I could tolerate and what I could not.

Troubleshooting tips that worked for me post-stoma surgery

- Take your time with food—try small amounts then chew thoroughly until the food is in liquid form in your mouth before you swallow. Remember, having a new stoma means that you have to start from scratch with discovering what you can and can't tolerate food-wise.
- Early on, I avoided eating fruits and vegetables with the skins on, tough and fibrous food, nuts, etc. Then very slowly started reintroducing them into my diet as my bowel healed.
- Drink a glass of water/liquid of choice after each meal—this helps the food move along in the gut.
- Don't force yourself to finish a meal—if you force yourself then you are pretty much guaranteed to make yourself sick!
- Sit upright while eating and for at least 30 minutes after each meal—this avoids blocking the path and movement of food making its way through the gut.
- Walk after every meal—I found this very effective in helping my gut with the digestion process. As you get stronger, you should try to walk as much as possible anyway to avoid developing deep vein thrombosis while in hospital.
- Try warm peppermint water or peppermint tea—it really helped me when I was feeling nauseated. Room temperature and warm liquids are friendlier to the gut I find.

- If you feel nauseated and off, it's ok if you skip a meal and stick to fluids. I think maintaining hydration is more important at this early stage, anyway.
- Take notice of your output! You really need to start paying attention to your stoma output post-surgery as it will indicate to you whether you are digesting certain foods properly or not. Having a stoma is truly like having a window into your gut. Passing wind is also a good sign that your new stoma is working early on.
- Just because you aren't tolerating or digesting certain foods immediately post-surgery, doesn't mean that you won't be able to tolerate them when your bowel is healed. Be patient with this!

Management of minor stoma blockages

I have had minor blockages of my stoma on several occasions. Helpful advice from my stoma nurses, combined with my own trial and error, has taught me how best to manage them when they happen. Apart from the blockage after my first surgery, I have never had another that severe and I have been able to manage them myself, at home.

My blockages (so far) have been caused by certain foods, which I call trigger foods. Please note: these will vary from person to person.

My trigger foods are:

- raw kale and cooked whole spinach/Asian greens?? (so weird)
- too much pineapple and mango
- Bircher muesli with high volumes of whole nuts and seeds
- coarsely shredded coconut/dried coconut chips or shards
- peas, corn, and whole enoki mushrooms
- quinoa increases my output volume dramatically and causes wind.

I prevent blockages from happening by:

- remaining upright for at least half an hour to an hour after eating
- moving after eating
- avoiding highly stringy foods like mangos and salads late in the evening or before bed
- chewing food well (this can be difficult to remember, depends how hungry I am)
- I really enjoy pineapple and mango. So, instead of cutting these trigger foods out of my diet completely; I try eating smaller portions or finely dicing them up. Putting them into smoothies is also good.

I experience the following signs and symptoms when I have a stoma blockage:

- nausea
- bloating
- my stoma swelling
- solid food ceases to pass into my bag
- sharp, intermittent abdominal pain as my bowel spasms.

Once I establish I have a block, I take the following steps:

- commence 24 hours of clear fluids until the blockage clears, increasing water intake while stoma is blocked
- have hot showers, alternating with ice pack application if stoma is swollen
- massage my abdomen, especially around the stoma
- maintain as much regular movement as possible, such as walking.

It is a good sign, once I notice solid foods starting to pass into the stoma bag. If I feel that the blockage has passed, I slowly introduce thicker foods into my diet i.e. soft pasta such as ravioli or tortellini, custard, well-cooked/pureed fruit and vegetables e.g. peeled & mashed or well-cooked potato/sweet potato, pureed apple without skins, plain banana smoothies etc.

Once I see that the thicker food is passing completely, I slowly go back onto my normal diet.

Important thing to note:

Do not rush into normal solids as your bowel will probably still be a little sluggish to digest, and make sure you chew your food well, walk after meals, and drink plenty of fluids.

NB: Please go to the hospital if:

- you are vomiting (especially if you are vomiting faecal matter)
- the stoma stops working completely
- the stoma colour turns from bright red to dusky
- you spike a temperature.

The art of balancing ileostomy output and maintaining adequate hydration

Despite having to avoid or modify how I consume certain foods containing fibre (such as the hard, stringy and difficult to digest types), I have found other types of fibre so important to my diet as they play a key role in managing my stoma output and also help control the amount of air I get in my bag.

You see, if I avoid fibre altogether and say, only eat protein (e.g. eggs, meats, etc.) and "white" carbs like white bread; my stoma output becomes too watery, food moves through my gut way too quickly impairing the ability to absorb nutrients. This causes the inconvenience of having to empty my bag way more often than usual and ultimately, can very quickly leave me dehydrated.

Conversely, if my stoma output becomes too thick to pass into my stoma bag, it can push my stoma back into my abdomen, causing the output to run underneath the base of my bag (where it sticks to my skin) and leak out, causing an awful, embarrassing mess. This has happened to me many times early on in my stoma journey, including while I was dining at an expensive restaurant in the city!

"Not too watery, not too thick" is the aim of the ileostomy game. Adequate sodium intake is also an essential element in maintaining appropriate levels of hydration.

I found what really works for me (with trial and error and sometimes by pure accident):

Cooked vegetables — are great at thickening my output, even better than fruit I find. This includes 'soft veggies' such as: broccoli, cauliflower, zucchini, sweet potato and pumpkin. If I don't eat vegetables regularly (I can be pretty naughty at times), my gut doesn't feel right. Adding veggies to casseroles in the slow cooker works well.

Chia seeds[37] — are most effective for me when they have been soaked. This was an accidental discovery after eating some chocolate chia cake. My output was nice and thick by the time it made its way through my gut. I found chia very gentle to the gut and bulked my output nicely because, when soaked, the seeds developed a thick gelatinous coating on them. Observing this is how I came to start making my "Gut-friendly Bircher"—recipe at the end of this chapter.

Natural/unsweetened plain Greek yogurt — this is something I consume regularly, in fact, pretty much every day (I use it in my Bircher). It really helps decrease the amount of gas emitted from my stoma and it works so well at neutralising odorous output caused by certain foods like eggs and fish.

Stewed/pureed fruit — such as apple is another ingredient I add into my Bircher. It thickens the output really well without making it too thick to pass into my bag.

Porridge — the funny thing with porridge is, if I eat it hot, immediately after making it, it doesn't really thicken my output. However, I found, by accident, that if I made a big batch of porridge and left it in the fridge, it became "gelatinous" and this thickened my output very effectively. I soak the oats for 1-2 days before I cook them with sultanas and spices, such as cinnamon and ginger, so it's flavoursome enough to eat cold. Maybe I am strange, but it works for me. To make it even thicker I sometimes add pre-soaked chia seeds after cooking the oats.

Slippery elm powder — I was advised to take this by a naturopath, and I have continued on with this periodically. It has properties said to soothe gut inflammation and digestion issues. When added to liquid, it creates a sludgy substance known as mucilage which thickens my output. **Note:** It has a mild, though not very nice, flavour, so I usually add it to my smoothies.

Psyllium capsules[38] — when I first got my stoma in 2011, the nurses gave me Metamucil (flavoured psyllium husk) powder to help thicken my output. I found that the psyllium in it was ground too finely for me and therefore would only thicken it slightly. I then bought coarser, unflavoured psyllium which I consumed for a few years in cereal and yoghurt, however the taste and the texture became really off-putting and eventually I couldn't stand having it. Thankfully, I discovered psyllium capsules before I went overseas on holidays one time. While travelling, I took two capsules with my meals (mostly breakfast and lunch) and it kept my output consistently thick and therefore I didn't have to empty my bag as often. This worked a treat while travelling because toilets weren't always easy to come by and I struggled with the lack of fibre in the food provided when holidaying. These capsules were a God send.

Sodium (salt) replacement — it is very important to be aware that those with ileostomies are more prone to becoming dehydrated, and quickly. This is due to no longer having the function of the large bowel to reabsorb fluids and salts back into the body. Dehydration can influence, but is not limited to: blood pressure, the function of the heart, and the function of your other organs, so it can be very dangerous. This is something I can take for granted and I forget to add extra salt to my meals at times. I need to pay more attention to this as I always seem to have very low-normal levels of sodium according to my blood tests. Luckily since having my stoma I crave salt way more than I did before my surgery, so this is my reminder to increase my intake. I try to add a bit of extra sea salt to every savoury meal. Sometimes, if I'm craving more salt, I snack on sea salt seasoned popcorn or salty haloumi cheese (obsessed), and I use oral electrolytes in the form of effervescent tablets added to a glass of water. Dehydration caused by sweating during exercise is an obvious one, but I can also feel quite dehydrated when I wake up in the morning. If I'm feeling a bit flat and nauseated on waking I will have an electrolyte drink. I also have electrolytes before and after exercise, otherwise I finish a gym class feeling lightheaded and nauseated—not just because I am unfit! The electrolyte tablets are another essential when travelling. **Please Note:** if you have kidney or heart issues please consult your doctor before consuming electrolyte products.

Natural ginger tablets for nausea — as a Crohnie, nausea can, and does, occur a lot, especially when travelling. I also suffer from pretty terrible motion sickness. Natural ginger tablets are a must when travelling as I find them very effective for relieving nausea, motion sickness, and general digestive pain. I started taking these as an alternative to conventional anti-nausea medication because I found that - most types cause me to have severe panic attacks and restlessness. No thanks!

My top tips for stoma management

- Always go with what feels right for you. Listen to your body and go with your gut! Pun may or may not be intended ;-)
- With a new stoma, take your time with your meals while your bowel is healing – chew thoroughly, have a full glass of water on hand, and walk after every meal.
- Always take extra stoma supplies (i.e. spare bag, seal, adhesive remover wipes, nappy bags, disposable wash cloths or wipes)

and perhaps even a change of clothes with you whenever you leave the house just in case you have an unexpected disaster when you are out. This is especially handy when your stoma is new and a little more unpredictable.

- It is very much trial and error with what works for you and in discovering what foods you can, or cannot, tolerate. For example, not all Crohn's sufferers are intolerant to gluten or dairy (I consume both), and no single diet will suit everyone.

- Everyone is different! One person's symptoms and tolerances/intolerances can differ vastly from another person's depending on where the Crohn's presents in the gastrointestinal tract and for many other reasons.

- Everyone has an opinion and is willing to give you advice. Just remember, something that might work for one person may not necessarily work for you. Listen to your gut regarding any advice that you receive. It's ok if you decide not to go with it! Do what's right for you.

- Dehydration is a real possibility, especially for those of us with ileostomies. Tune into your body and check in with how you are feeling regarding symptoms of dehydration (especially on waking, on hot days, before/during/after exercise or when sick with fever) and if you are feeling off, replace your salts ASAP!

Bonus Bite!

During bag change, I like to tuck a nappy bag into my pants with the opening directly below my stoma so that when I take my bag off, my output doesn't shoot out all over me and the floor (which has happened many times before). It's not effective 100% of the time, but it has definitely avoided many accidents.

Meagan's Stoma-friendly Bircher

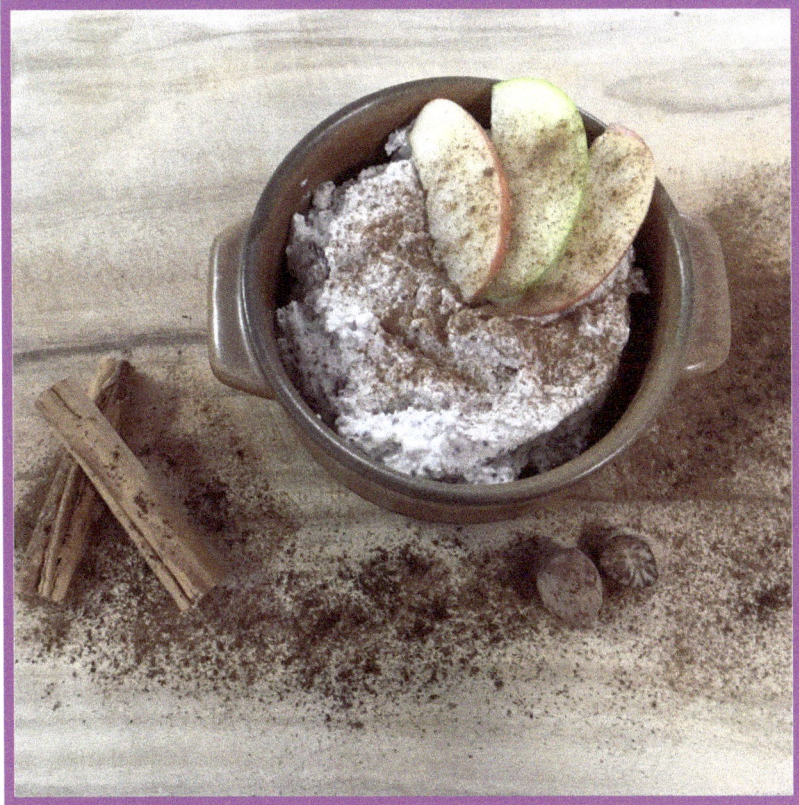

After working out what foods agreed with me, I created this gut-friendly breakfast recipe (specific to me), as eating conventional Bircher would often result in a stoma blockage. I like to make up a big batch for the week and have it on hand in the fridge because it saves time and prevents me stressing about what I will make for breakfast every morning. I find Bircher tastes even better with time because this allows the spices and flavours to permeate through the mixture. The mixture will last as long as the expiry date on the natural yoghurt. This recipe is great too because you can modify it to how you like it.

Ingredients:

- 7 stewed apples with skins on (Leaving the skins on does not upset my gut. I cook the apples until soft and mushy in a saucepan with a dash of apple cider vinegar, a dash of water and ground ginger, cinnamon, vanilla and nutmeg to taste)
- 5 tablespoons of chia seeds
- 5 tablespoons of ground nut meal with skins (I often alternate between hazelnut and almond meal)
- 2/3 cup raw and uncooked oats
- 1 litre natural unsweetened or Greek yoghurt
- Handful of sultanas
- Ground cinnamon and vanilla (or whatever spices you wish you use).

Method:

1. Pre-cook apples and allow to cool somewhat before adding to the mixture.
2. While cooking the apples, add all other ingredients into a large air-tight container.
3. Mix all ingredients thoroughly.
4. Allow the mixture to sit in the fridge for a couple of hours or overnight before eating.

Meagan's Stoma-friendly Chia Porridge

Ingredients:

- 3 cups Milk of choice (coconut, nut milk, dairy)
- 1-1.5 cups Raw rolled oats
- Following spices adjusted to taste:
  - Grated whole nutmeg
  - Ground cinnamon
  - Ground black pepper
  - Ground turmeric
  - Ground vanilla bean
  - Ground or freshly grated ginger
  - Fresh ground fennel seeds
  - Ground cardamom
  - A couple of whole Cloves or 1 drop doTerra clove oil
  - 1-2 cinnamon quills if desired.
- 2 tablespoons of chia seeds
- Handful of sultanas/grated or precooked apple for sweetness if desired.

Method:

1. I soak approx. 1 cup – 1.5 cup oats in enough water to cover with a pinch of salt overnight
2. As well as soaking the oats, I steep the chai spices in approx. 3 cups of milk of choice overnight. I often use coconut or almond milk.

3. So, to the three cups of milk, or, enough to cover the oats when it's time to cook them, I add:

   1-2 teaspoons (or adjust to taste) of:
   - Grated whole nutmeg
   - Ground cinnamon
   - Ground black pepper
   - Ground turmeric
   - Ground vanilla bean
   - Ground or freshly grated ginger

   ½- 1 teaspoons (or adjust to taste) of:
   - Fresh ground fennel seeds
   - Ground cardamom
   - 1 drop of doTerra clove oil.

   Sometimes I add:
   - A drop each of DoTerra cinnamon, black pepper, ginger and cardamom oil
   - Or, a couple of whole cinnamon quills.

4. Steep spices in milk maximum overnight. I wouldn't recommend leaving for a couple of nights it makes it too bitter.
5. Next day strain oats soaking in water and remove cinnamon quills/anything else inedible if added from the milk.
6. Add oats to the milk. **
7. Cook the oats/sultanas/apple in the milk and continue stirring until it becomes creamy porridge.
8. While the oats are cooking, I soak 2 tablespoons of chia seeds in some of the milk until they develop the gelatinous coating. Add the chia to the oats when cooked.

** For sweetness: I also like to add a handful of sultanas and grated apple to the mix, or, I pre-cook the diced apples in cinnamon, nutmeg, vanilla, a dash of apple cider vinegar and a dash of water until tender and add the apples to the cooked porridge.

PART TWO

SKIN ISSUES & MANAGEMENT

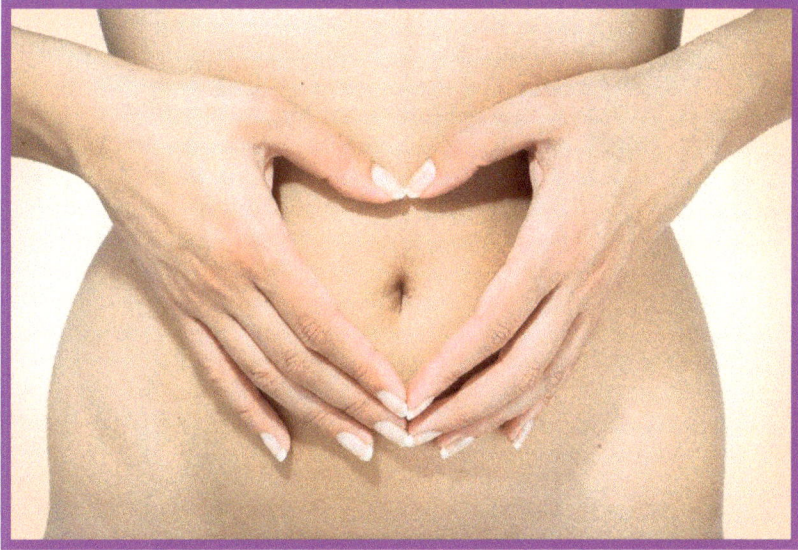

The skin is the largest organ of the body. Normally healthy skin helps us to keep our body hydrated, provides a barrier to protect the body from pathogens[39] in the environment, and has a certain amount of elasticity to allow for growth and movement of the body. These examples are only the tip of the iceberg regarding the functions of our skin.

It's only when you develop skin conditions (such as, like me, dermatitis and psoriasis) where the skin's function has been compromised, that you realise how important our skin actually is. If the skin is compromised by these conditions, I have found that helping the skin retain moisture and elasticity is key.

Although the skin needs a certain amount of moisture, it does not do well if it's constantly sitting in excess moisture, i.e. wearing non-breathable underwear, not drying yourself properly after a shower/swim, etc.

So, what is psoriasis?

"Psoriasis… occurs when skin cells grow too quickly.

The result can be seen as inflamed, thickened and scaly areas of skin.
It can also affect other areas, such as the finger or toenails. In some cases,
the person may also have sore and inflamed joints at the same time.
When this occurs, it is called psoriatic arthritis.
Psoriasis is not an infection and is not contagious… it is caused by over-
activity of your body's immune system. The extra inflammation makes
the skin cells grow and multiply too quickly.
The body is not able to shed these excess skin cells, so they pile up on the
surface of the skin…"
There's no specific cause of psoriasis, but the condition can often be
triggered by stress (like many chronic illnesses), skin injury, medications,
and hormone changes or imbalances. (Psoriasis Australia)

The link between Crohn's disease and psoriasis

It's very interesting to note that there is research out there that supports the link between psoriasis and Crohn's disease. According to one source, psoriasis very commonly coexists in patients with inflammatory bowel disease.

"…findings from gene and molecular research may explain the
connection. Scientists have long known that psoriasis and Crohn's disease
have a number of polymorphisms (genetic mutations) in common…
The same genes that make a person susceptible to psoriasis may also make
that person susceptible to Crohn's…" (National Psoriasis Foundation)

How psoriasis & skin issues have affected my life
Genital psoriasis

According to DermNet NZ, *"Genital psoriasis affects the genital skin, which includes the pubic area, vulva or penis, skin folds and buttocks. It affects adults as well as children…Genital skin can also be affected in inverse or **flexural psoriasis**, i.e. psoriasis that mainly affects the skin* *folds. Genital psoriasis may be associated with considerable discomfort and embarrassment and may severely impair the quality of life and sexual well-being of those affected".*

This has been an ongoing problem for me for a number of years now. At the time of diagnosis, I had developed chronic splitting of the vulvar and perianal areas to the point that even wiping with toilet paper would tear my skin. This was extremely painful. I could also peel strips of my skin off like it was snakeskin. It was very disabling, embarrassing and it drastically impacted my self-esteem and sex life.

The only management options I was given by various dermatologists[40] were steroid creams. After significant trial and error, I ceased using them not only due to the long-term side effects they can cause, but more positively, I had finally figured out what worked for me. It obviously hasn't cured the condition, but it has allowed me to manage the condition very well on a daily basis.

Management Tips

In my opinion, based on my personal experience, I find drying the area well and regularly moisturising (at least daily after showers) are the keys to managing this type of psoriasis.

Steroid creams, especially those formulated at a higher dose, are intended for thicker skin exposed to the elements. They are very bad for the genital area as they thin the skin after a period of time and can exacerbate the splitting associated with this condition.

I only use water to clean the genital and buttock area. This includes avoiding shower gel, soap or perfumed cleansers as they can irritate the condition.

My usual evening routine after a shower:
- I gently pat the genital and buttock area dry with a clean towel. I avoid rubbing the area vigorously to dry.
- I use a hairdryer on the cool setting to dry these areas as much as possible.

- Once the skin feels dry, I apply only a small amount of appropriate (natural/hypoallergenic/gentle) moisturiser formulated for these sensitive areas (I use the brand <u>Hope's Relief Premium eczema cream</u>: it contains a high proportion of botanical ingredients, it's low in preservative, safe for the genital area, safe for babies, it's also fast absorbing and non-greasy). Remember to patch test first before you use a new product. And try to keep the cream away from your openings. The genital mucosa is very similar to the mucosa in your mouth.
- I apply a small amount of <u>Lucas' Papaw Ointment</u> to my bottom crease (especially to the sinus opening where my anus was), making sure it is spread along the crease. This creates a protective barrier for the skin and helps lock in the moisturiser. I then ensure it is rubbed in well so that there's no excess ointment sitting on the skin.

Managing chronic splits in my perianal skin

I found that <u>Cavilon barrier wipes or spray</u> helped to heal the skin well and prevented further splits from developing.

Post-shower, I would do my usual regime with the hairdryer and moisturiser. But I would then apply the Cavilon followed by the hairdryer again to dry, or set, the Cavilon so a protective film was formed over the split and surrounding skin.

Some other helpful ideas:
- I wear loose-fitting, breathable underwear such as cotton briefs so sweat doesn't get trapped in the area as much.
- I avoid wearing underwear to bed most nights to let the areas air. Cotton boxers are good for this.
- I change out of wet swimming costumes as soon as I can after being in the pool.
- During my period, to avoid the skin sitting in menstrual blood for a prolonged time, I use a <u>Juju menstrual cup</u>. Pre-

vious to the cup I was using tampons. I found the menstrual blood would break down my skin and split my vulvar skin if I used a pad.

- When I have splits in this skin, urination can really sting, the same goes when wiping with toilet paper. When I "wipe", I actually just hold the toilet paper to the area instead of using the wiping action.

Sex is another difficult and highly painful endeavour as the friction can tear the skin or make any existing splits worse, even bleed. I have had very deep splits and subsequent bleeding after sex that have taken a long time to heal. To try to reduce this from happening, I use a natural lubricant (I use the brand Sylk) during sex. This has greatly helped in protecting my skin and made my experiences much more enjoyable.

Psoriasis on my knuckles

Up until recently, I have suffered from contact dermatitis over my hands on and off for many years. My hands would develop blisters that would bust and become weepy and my skin would be furiously itchy. After the weeping stopped, my hands would dry out and I would develop deep and painful cracks that would bleed, especially in my knuckles. Back then this was treated as any other psoriasis, with steroid creams and ointments.

A few years back, I started developing warts over my hands. The highest concentration of warts was found over my knuckles of my right hand. I went to a skin clinic and the doctor there proceeded to freeze the warts off. The burns from this were so extensive that I developed a massive blister over my knuckles.

Being a nurse, I couldn't wear gloves or wash with the harsh soaps due to the pain. The compromised skin on my hands, and difficulty with hand washing, put me at risk of germ exposure and also of transmission to others. After the blister healed, I developed scarring and a dry scale over the area. It would often become red, itchy, cracked and peel.

I felt so embarrassed at work with patient contact and shaking people's hands and people would often ask me what was wrong with my hand. To my dismay, I was diagnosed with localised psoriasis that would continue to interfere with my nursing work and cause problems for many years to come. I found the steroid cream prescribed to me by my dermatologist at the time made my skin peel more and impaired the skin from healing, so I decided to stop using it. This is where trial and error came in until I found what worked for me in the form of essential oils.

I can happily share, after significant experimentation, my winning oil combination to manage the psoriasis on my knuckles! Today, it's so well managed that people wouldn't even know I have psoriasis.

Management Tips

- Mix 4 drops each of: <u>Doterra</u> clary sage, lavender, frankincense and tea tree oil into a small container of <u>soft white paraffin</u> and apply to knuckles/other psoriasis areas on the hands after a shower at night, just before bed.
- The key to managing this condition is daily application, even if it looks better, and avoid peeling the dry skin off.
- I always wear rubber gloves while doing the dishes because the dish liquid can irritate the skin.
- I avoid perfumed moisturisers at all costs because they can sting and flare my skin up.

Peristomal (the skin around the stoma) psoriasis

Developing psoriasis under the stoma bag was a challenging time for me. The psoriasis developed from a burn on my skin from my stoma output after it leaked. The red, itchy and painful sore eventually spread around the whole area under my stoma bag.

It turned into a horrible sequence of red sores > dry scaly skin > I would (foolishly) peel the skin off > the skin would become weepy and infected > the open skin would react to the adhesive on the bag > my bag wouldn't stick to my skin. A terrible, vicious cycle.

I tried so many different creams and ointments, but they didn't really help or they prevented the bag from sticking to my skin. I honestly didn't think that I was ever going to get better. But one day I remembered I had left over steroid cream from the time I had been referred to a dermatologist for my genital psoriasis. I started to blow dry the skin on a cool setting at the time of changing my bag and applied a little of the cream to my skin after it was dry and it seemed to reduce the inflammation.

With this information, I again went back to the dermatologist. I had a punch biopsy taken to ensure it was psoriasis (which it was). I didn't feel that I got a lot of guidance from that particular dermatologist, so I got referred to another one. He prescribed a particular steroid ointment rather than a cream, which absorbed so much better into my skin and didn't interfere with my bag sticking to my skin properly. Gradually with daily maintenance, the skin healed and I have not had a flare up in that area since!

Management Tips

To heal my peristomal psoriasis:
- When washing and drying the area, I was very gentle – only using patting motions as being vigorous hurts and damages the skin.
- At every bag change, after cleaning the skin with water, I blow-dried (on a cool setting) the skin around the stoma until it felt dry.
- I avoided peeling the skin off!
- Next, I applied the steroid ointment sparingly on the red lesions in a very small circular motion until absorbed.

- I applied the bag and held it against my skin longer than usual so the heat would help the bag stick better.
- I used the steroid ointment for as long as the dermatologist advised me. It really didn't take long for the skin to heal in this instance.

My usual daily routine since the psoriasis has healed

I have continued to use the gentle washing and drying technique to maintain healthy, intact skin and I have incorporated using the blow dryer on the skin around the stoma with each daily bag change (after cleaning and hand drying the skin) ever since. This helps prevent damp skin from breaking down and causing a reoccurrence of psoriasis. Happy to say it hasn't returned since that one time (so far).

Bag Removal Sequence

Here's another tip for during bag removal. I use this to avoid vigorous rubbing of the skin around my stoma bag. I use <u>Welland Adhesive remover wipes</u> to dissolve the sticky residue from around the bag.

After you tear open the sachet, pour a little water into the sachet then pour the solution directly where the skin and the bag meet.

This allows me to gently ease the bag off little by little rather than having to pull it off the skin which can irritate. Once I have the bag free of my skin, I use the wipe itself to remove the remaining adhesive from the exposed skin.

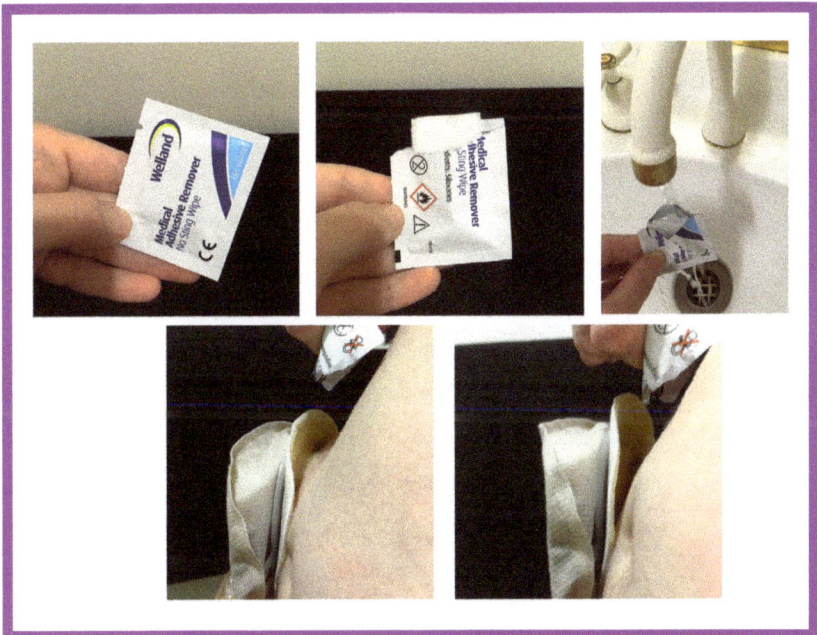

Psoriasis of the navel

Psoriasis in my belly button has been, along with periorificial dermatitis, one of the most stubborn conditions to get under control. I have been suffering with this the longest. My poor belly button dries out, splits, bleeds, weeps, gets infected and smelly, and becomes very uncomfortable.

The situation was not helped by the fact I use a belt around my lower waist to keep my stoma in place which can cover up the belly button at times and prevent the air getting to it. I also have a lot of scarring from my two bowel surgeries and a punch biopsy there, so the skin isn't what it used to be.

I have tried a lot of remedies for this condition also, and for a while, it seemed like nothing was going to work. However, after extensive trial and error (what a surprise), I have finally found products and a routine that has kept the navel skin under control!

Management Tips

- After my nightly shower, I use a cotton tip very gently to dry the area and remove any gunk from it. If I'm too rough with the cotton tip it can split my belly button skin and make it bleed – ouch!
- I follow up the cotton tip with a blow dryer on the cold setting to help dry it properly.
- Avoid peeling the dry skin off!
- Gently apply a thin layer of Hope's Relief Premium eczema cream to the belly button with a cotton tip and rub the excess in with my finger until absorbed. I would even apply over the peeling skin, being careful not to accidentally tear it off completely.
- As a protective barrier, I then apply a very thin layer of Lucas' Papaw Ointment over the top with a cotton tip and rub in the

excess with my finger again. This helps keep the moisturiser locked into the skin.

- Moisture is key but you don't want to drown the skin in cream and ointment because this will be too hard for the skin to absorb and will eventually break the area down.
- I apply my stoma bag with the belt loops diagonally (pictured below) so that the belt sits underneath my belly button to allow for airflow.
- Again, continued daily application, even when it looks better, will give you the best results.

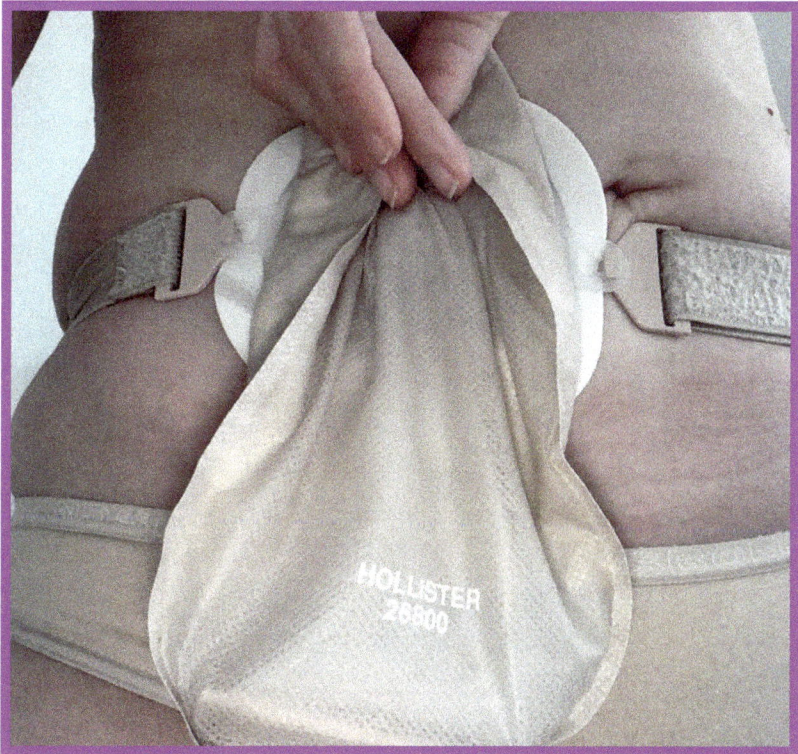

Periorificial dermatitis

"Periorificial dermatitis is a common facial skin problem characterised by groups of itchy or tender small red papules. It is given this name because the papules occur around the eyes, the nostrils, the mouth and occasionally, the genitals." (DermNet NZ)

This particular problem has been up there with genital psoriasis as one of the most deeply embarrassing and painful conditions I have endured and it affected my confidence severely. The facial rash has flared up about 3 or 4 times to date.

Each time, the skin around my nostrils, mouth and eyes would start to develop red lumps similar to pimples, which would eventually break out into red and dry scaly skin and spread over my face in the shape of an oxygen mask. It would become so raw and painful that it would hurt to eat and sting when applying moisturiser. Nothing would soothe it.

So far, I have found the following things responsible for flaring up this condition:

- using sunscreen on the face
- drinking caffeinated coffee (a theory of mine but still not 100% on this though)
- swimming in a chlorinated pool
- stress certainly doesn't help either.

I was at my wit's end trying to figure out what would get rid of this, so I went to a dermatologist about it. He prescribed steroid ointments and immunosuppressing creams formulated for the face. I tried these but they irritated the skin and made the inflammation rebound even more. I stopped using these products immediately because they were just not helping whatsoever.

I tried so many different remedies, including:

- prednisone tablets - worked while I took them, then flared up terribly after a few days of stopping

- making a slippery elm paste to apply to my face - which did nothing
- bathing the face with warm saltwater - which dried my face out even more
- applying essential oils - which irritated the skin more
- trialling different moisturisers for sensitive skin - which again stung and irritated the face.

At this stage, I stopped using moisturisers!

I also stopped exfoliating my face in the hope it would get rid of the inflamed and scaly skin. Stopped wearing makeup and using anything else that might irritate the skin. I really had to dial back what I was using on my face and go with the bare basics. The only thing that I could tolerate was <u>soft white paraffin</u>.

I was at work, desperate for answers, one day when a fellow nurse told me she had started using wet wraps[41] for the eczema on her son's legs and it had worked brilliantly. It made me start thinking how I could adapt this principle to my face rash. The methods I developed did help eventually. However, unfortunately, in this situation, I have found that time is the main predictor for the skin healing. Patience and repetition is key!

Management Tips

- My best friends have been a clean washcloth and soft white paraffin during each flare up.
- I avoided peeling the dry skin off or exfoliating.
- Twice daily, I would saturate the washcloth in very warm water and hold it on my face, and then very gently pat it over the sore areas. The warm water was so soothing to my face.
- After using the washcloth, I would pat the face softly with a dry towel but avoid drying my face completely, leaving it slightly damp.

- In the mornings—after slightly dampening my face, I would apply a very thin layer of white soft paraffin over the sore areas, careful not to make it too thick because it looked weird going to work with a shiny face.
- In the evenings—after slightly dampening my face, I would apply thickish layers of white soft paraffin over the sore areas to act like a barrier. I did not rub this in but let it sit on top of the skin to help protect it overnight.
- I maintained this routine until my face healed. I really think this process helped the skin to heal and renew underneath the layer of paraffin. During this time, I avoided swimming in chlorine, wearing makeup, drinking coffee, wearing sunscreen on my face and any other triggers I had discovered. When my face healed, I slowly introduced a moisturiser and a very gentle and mild exfoliator back into my routine. I patch tested these products at first because I was scared it would irritate my skin again but they ended up being well tolerated.

My usual routine when my skin isn't flared up:
- Every morning I wash my face thoroughly with plain tap water.
- I use Moogoo Natural Skin Milk Udder Cream daily on my face after a shower at night and paraffin as needed on the dry bits, especially in the creases either side of my nose.
- I exfoliate once or twice a week depending how dry my face feels or before I apply makeup. I only use a block of pure French white clay – applying it to a wet face at the start of my shower. I allow it to dry over the face while showering and then use a washcloth to gently remove the clay. This routine leaves my skin feeling very soft and smooth. I avoid using an exfoliating glove or rough vigorous movements because, you guessed it, it may irritate the skin.

My top 3 tips for skin issue management

- I have found that the key to managing my psoriasis/skin related conditions is consistent daily treatment, even when the skin looks better.
- Avoid peeling off the dry skin. I know it is tempting to pull it off but I have found that leaving the dry skin intact protects the new skin underneath. When I used to peel the dry skin off (especially in my belly button and under my stoma bag), it would make my skin weep and become raw and painful. This ultimately prevents the skin from healing.
- Less is more! Moisturising is key, but you don't want to drown the skin in cream and ointment because this will be too hard for the skin to absorb and it will eventually break the area down.

PART THREE

PELVIC & PERIANAL ISSUE MANAGEMENT

Management of various perianal problems

At the time of my diagnosis and early on (prior to my stoma bag surgery), I suffered from a painful perianal ulcer, a large skin tag and multiple anal fissures. I was in a tremendous amount of pain from even the simplest of things, such as coughing, sneezing, getting up out of my seat, sitting down and/or bending over—it was just torture.

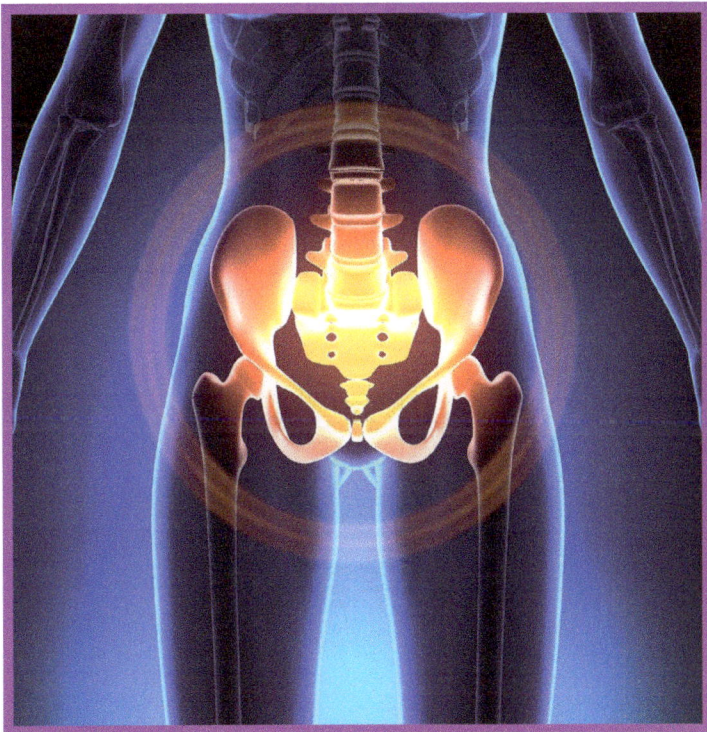

Not to mention the painful anal spasms[42], bleeding, and the residual stool that would ooze (when the spasms released) into my underwear after every bowel movement. My life was pain, discomfort, disgust and embarrassment.

However, at this time, my surgeon and treating doctors suggested things that really helped and decreased my pain levels while enabling me to keep my perianal area feeling cleaner. Some of these techniques are still very useful to this day. The other things I just worked out as I went.

They have helped me deal with the complications that arose from surgery in 2013, including, chronic drainage from the perianal sinus, that used to be my anus, would mean excess moisture was constantly sitting around my bottom. As well as, my most recent, and bizarre, complication (in 2018), where a second sinus opened up in my bottom and began draining - yes, I had two butt holes! You have to laugh, well, maybe not at the time, but I can now ;-)

Anal spasms: treat the spasm, treat the pain

I was prescribed <u>Rectogesic ointment</u>[43] to apply to my anus when the spasming occurred. This relaxed the sphincter muscles and decreased the spasm and the associated pain. The only side effect was a slight headache with each use. Paracetamol and other pain killers do not work for this problem as the spasm is what causes the pain! *Treat the spasm, treat the pain.*

And speaking of pain, during flare-ups, I would get terrible pain in my lower back and tail bone area that was so uncomfortable I couldn't sleep. I found that having a shower as hot as I could stand and running the water directly onto my back would relieve the pain so much that I didn't need pain medication and the best result was some much-needed sleep.

Anal discharge: baby wipes

I was advised by a doctor at the time to use baby wipes when the ooze occurred. I found this was way better than toilet paper because it was thicker and didn't fall apart or stick to my bottom. It was moist so it cleaned the area more effectively. I used to carry pocket-sized wipes with me everywhere at this time. I also used to use panty liners to prevent the ooze from soaking through my underwear.

Discharge leakage prevention: makeup pads

Due to the constant ooze from my bottom, I was sick of my underwear being soaked by the discharge and staining my clothes. I started placing round cotton makeup pads folded in half into my bottom crease to soak up the excess discharge. This helped protect the perianal skin and prevented it from going onto my underwear. I still do this now and carry spare pads with me everywhere I go. Just change them as needed. If the discharge is heavier, I place two makeup pads, layered together, in the bottom crease.

When I had my multiple rectal drains in place to try to clear the pelvic infection, I still had ooze occurring around the drain site. I also used makeup pads for this – I cut a slit into the pad and placed it around the drain at the entrance of my bottom so that my skin was protected from the discharge.

Decreasing pain caused by anal wounds: salt baths

I still swear by <u>Sitz (salt) baths</u>[44] for my bottom whenever I need to soothe pain and clean the area. Dissolve a teaspoon of table salt in a Sitz tub (pictured on following page) of warm water.

Sit in the water for approximately 10-15 minutes. Then refill the tub with just plain warm water and sit in it for another 5 minutes to rid the area of salt which can be quite drying on my skin. This process

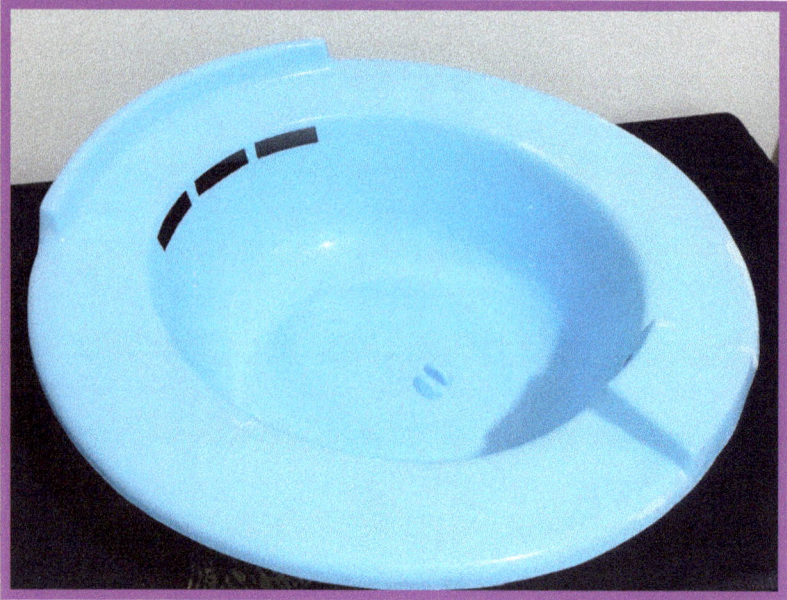

helps facilitate the drainage of muck from the bottom, manages infection and eases pain. I continue to do this until the pain and/or infection is resolved.

Bonus Bite!

Obviously, you can't bring a sitz basin with you travelling. When I found myself faced with this issue, I got the idea of using something I already had in the house, though it was for an entirely different issue, a nasal and sinus wash bottle (pictured on following page).

It's got a straw and a nozzle and comes with sachets of a salt/bicarb mix. Pour warm water into the bottle, pour in the contents of the sachet, and shake to dissolve. Then while you're showering it's a good way to gently clean your bottom wound as the warm water comes out in a steady stream each time you squeeze the bottle and you can direct the stream into the right position in the bottom crease. It's pretty effective and better than nothing while you're travelling!

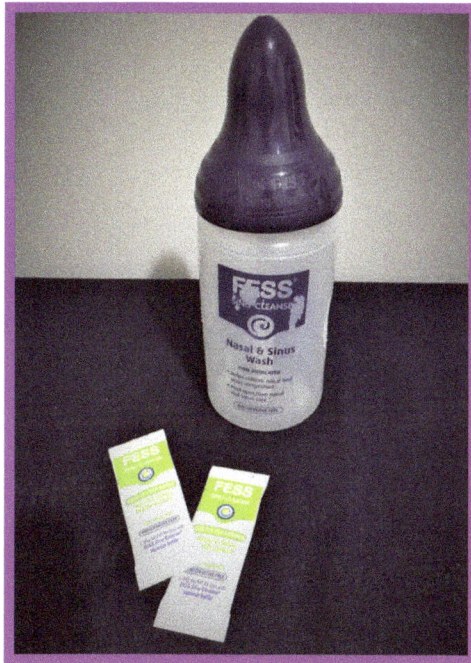

Pubic pustules

This was yet another heavy and painful period of my life. I started developing infected pustules[45] over my pubic skin, possibly folliculitis[46]. It would cause such pain and nausea with terrible swelling in the skin over the pubic bone and a discharge of pus. I remember getting the sweats and almost fainting one day because I knocked the inflamed area on a table corner. At one stage I ended up with approximately six pustules at the same time! I saw a dermatologist and my colorectal surgeon about this issue, but they didn't seem to know what they were or how to advise me regarding management. I started doing my own research about similar conditions and worked out how to heal these pustules using multiple remedies. Happy to report this problem hasn't occurred since.

Management Tips

- I washed the area daily with <u>pHisohex Anti-bacterial Wash</u> to help kill the bacteria causing the infection.
- I made sure the shower water was as hot as I could stand and applied a hot compress to the area (I just used a washcloth soaked in hot water).
- In the shower under the hot water I would gently squeeze to see if pus would come out. Releasing the pus was a big relief regarding pain management. The heat helps with inflammation and opening the pores, releasing pus.
- After a shower, I would apply a sparing amount of <u>Otocomb Otic Ointment</u> (a combination of steroid medication and antibiotics. This is a prescription-only medication) directly on the pustules. I did this twice daily until they were healed.
- I avoided shaving or clipping this area
- My usual routine once the area healed:
- I continue to avoid shaving or clipping the area and instead have the hair removed by "<u>Sugaring</u>[47]".
- I regularly exfoliate the area to avoid ingrown hairs and folliculitis.

PART FOUR

STRESS & ANXIETY

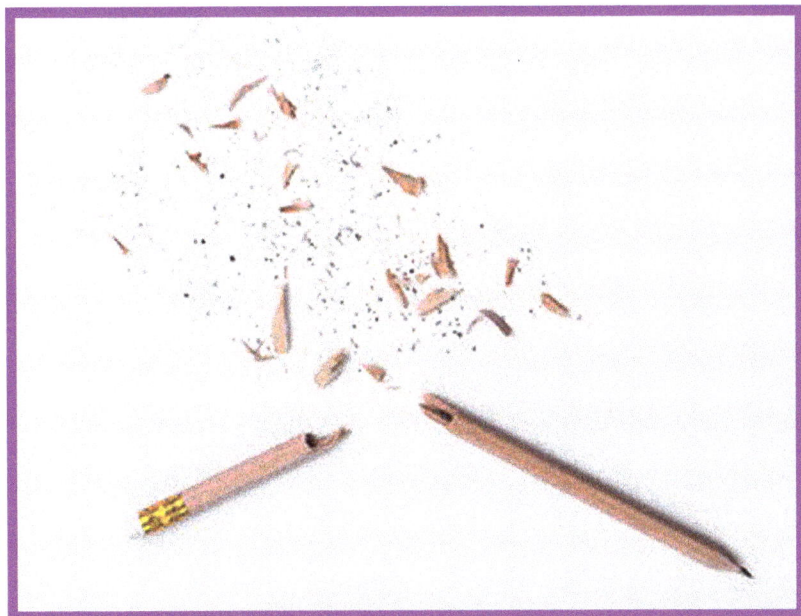

S tress and anxiety are major influences on your health! I have personally experienced their direct effects too often to ignore the connection. I noticed how they flare up my psoriasis, the inflammation in my gut and the rest of my body as well as slowing my recovery time.

I believe regular stress management is key for anyone suffering with chronic illness and the associated anxiety and depression.

Stress influences so many factors, including:

- sleep quality
- the stability of blood glucose levels
- inflammation
- the immune system
- weight gain or loss
- the ability to focus on and complete tasks properly
- it diminishes feelings of accomplishment and erodes your self-esteem.

Basically, stress influences your overall mental, physical, and spiritual health and outlook on life.

I have experienced anxiety throughout most of my life. From being paranoid about having a terminal illness and experiencing OCD behaviours in my early years (pre-Crohn's diagnosis), to reaching the peak of my anxiety in 2015 when I experienced continuous panic attacks for a whole weekend.

In 2015, I presented myself to the mental health department at my local hospital and there began my journey to recovery. I did end up taking anti-depressants as a desperate last resort and only after intense and lengthy discussions with the mental health doctor.

What stuck with me the most from this experience were the words of the clinical nurse looking after me that day, he said, "The symptoms of your anxiety (the sweating, the pounding heart, the nausea and vomiting) won't kill you. The more you try to repress these feelings, the stronger the anxiety will fight back. Just acknowledge that they are there and let them do their worst. They won't hurt you."

This was the lightbulb moment for me! I felt free knowing that these thoughts and physical manifestations couldn't harm me, that I didn't have to buy into them, that thoughts are not fact and I was still in control of my mind. I was finally free from the unending, exhausting fight I was fighting.

After that, I gradually got better, and my panic attacks stopped. I still feel a bit anxious at times, but it doesn't scare me anymore. I have the tools to manage it. I also feel stronger and less fearful because of my experiences and for that I am grateful.

In my opinion, and experience, taking a pill alone without actively undertaking the personal development process will not help you achieve sustainable lifelong stability. I am very grateful that as a registered nurse I was armed with this knowledge. I knew that my recovery would take work and would need to continue throughout my lifetime. I also tried not to look at taking the antidepressants with a timeframe in mind of when I would wean off them. I just had to accept that recovery would take as long as it would take.

Getting control of your stress and anxiety involves daily work to start to create new thinking patterns and practices. Practicing gratitude is a very powerful way of changing your negative perspective through acknowledging and celebrating the positives (however big or small) and the good that we experience each day – things that we usually take for granted. Personally, this has really flipped my thinking around!

Management and maintenance of stress for me involves:

- journaling my thoughts and feelings
- keeping a daily gratitude diary
- reading self-development books
- listening to music and dancing around the house when I wash the dishes, cook and clean
- attending painting classes
- attending a regular yoga class
- having warm showers (they always calm me down)
- practicing meditation and mindfulness - I use a meditation app, but also just sit and count my breaths, or notice something in nature with one or more of my senses
- taking time for myself as often as possible
- sitting in my happy place: my local waterfront.

I have also been seeing a life coach since 2014 to keep me on track and accountable for my actions and the intentions that I set. I am a huge believer in the power of self-development and growth, as in, owning your shit and working on it.

If you harbour the negative without sitting with the feelings, working through them and releasing them, how are you able to create the space for more positivity and calm in your life?

This has been me—so totally stressed and unhappy in my job for the last number of years that it started manifesting as new physical and mental health issues. I wanted to walk out so many times in the middle of my shift. I honestly felt, and feel, that doing work that I don't derive purpose and joy from eats away at my soul.

My body was really being tested and looking back I can now see how badly I had minimised my physical and mental health again. That it took a painful new health issue, developing a second perianal sinus, to make me decide to take leave from work so I could try to formulate a new career plan.

It took me eight weeks to feel like I was gaining back some control over my health and to feel like I could, and would, pursue a new career path - something true to me. Since my time off, my psoriasis has come under control, the second perianal sinus has closed over, I have weaned off my antidepressant (I will admit there has been some bumps in the road with this) and I have almost completed writing this book.

I won't lie though, taking on this journey has at times felt overwhelming and, on many occasions, I've felt lost with regards to where I was heading in life. I know I am not perfect and try to not have unrealistic, perfect expectations of myself. Even with everything I have learnt on my journey, I still have to remind myself to continue to manage my stress levels and make decisions true to myself and that align with my health. That said...

Do I still go to bed far too late, far too often?

Yes!

Do I have big nights on alcohol at times?

Yes!

Do I still have massive junk food binges at times?

Yes!

Do I lack motivation at times?

Yes!

Are there periods of time (sometimes weeks)
where I just can't be bothered meditating, etc?

Yes!

Do I go into negative thought spirals at times?

Yes!

Do I get fed up with my time-consuming self-care regime
(my daily skin and perianal management process) at times?

Yes!

Am I human?

Yes!

I think it's important to mention that the stress, and its direct impact on my self-esteem and health, that comes with beating myself up about everything in the list above, is exactly why practicing patience with myself and self-acceptance is so vital!

Not only does it aid in influencing me to make decisions aligned with my health and truth, but also in managing my overall daily stress levels.

Guilt is not useful…for anyone!

Time to let it go!

PART FIVE

LEARNING TO ADVOCATE FOR YOURSELF

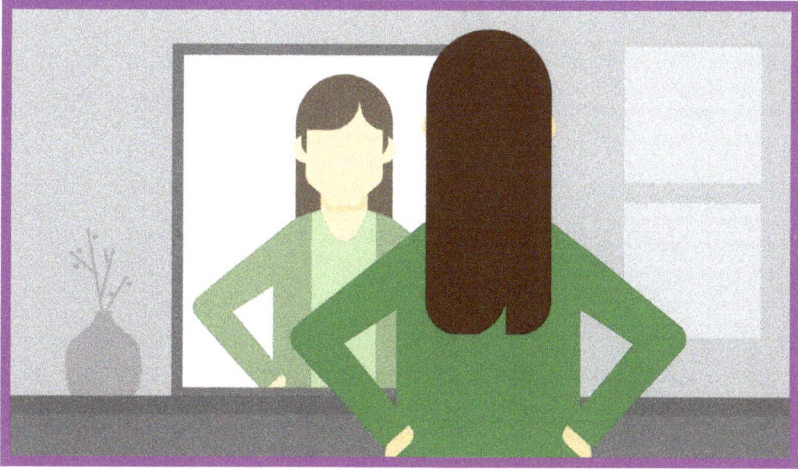

Early on I was too scared to speak up or ask too many questions as I feared being thought of as a difficult patient or a 'know it all' by the medical professionals. Especially with me being a registered nurse. I was worried that it would negatively influence their treatment of me.

Instead of feeling empowered, I felt scared and defeated. So, what changed? I got fed up.

This internal shift happened during a time where I was having a lot of problems with myositis and a Crohn's flare-up due to not being able to take my biologic medication. While this was happening, I was attending numerous hospital appointments, seeing different junior doctors each time, who had to familiarise themselves with my history and current issue every - single - time!!

I would have to take time off work to get to the hospital, sit for hours in the waiting room to then have a 20-minute max appointment ending with the doctor, through no fault of their own, saying that they would have to talk to the specialist as they did not know how to manage this issue. I was so angry that I was continually wasting my time and theirs, that I was losing pay from missing work, and that I didn't have an effective management plan in place while I was so sick.

My emotions got the better of me one day and I actually complained to the last junior doctor I saw about how fed up I was over my time being wasted. I was met with such empathy and understanding, and that doctor actually wrote a letter about this to my GP. I was still infuriated when I got home and directly emailed my gastroenterologist about it myself.

What happened then?

My gastroenterologist put into place that I was to only see him at appointments from then on. This allowed for continuity and greater expertise in managing this issue. He then referred me to a neurologist, where I received my muscular dystrophy carrier gene diagnosis; I was placed back onto Humira, and for some time, control was gained over my Crohn's that had gone rogue in the interim.

This really hit home to me that I had to be assertive and take control of my own health and self-advocate for my own sake if I wasn't happy about my management or care. I really needed to speak up because no one else was going to do it for me. I couldn't imagine what would have happened if I didn't assert myself that day?!

From then on, I have continued to speak up assertively (not aggressively) if I have an issue or concern because at the end of the day, it's MY HEALTH and QUALITY OF LIFE we are talking about (and yours)! I love that there is a lesson to learn with each 'negative' event that is encountered, and I am grateful for that.

Tips on how to assert yourself more

See a GP who you have a great rapport with, who listens to you, takes your complaints seriously and follows things up without hesitation. My GP is amazing!

When approaching medical staff, be firm, not aggressive: it's important that the medicos listen to us, but they are not there to be attacked. (To put this into perspective, think about how you feel when approached aggressively or when you feel attacked!)

To feel empowered regarding your health and its management, having all of your questions and concerns answered by your medical team is very important: Write down a list of questions when going into an appointment or when they see you on their ward rounds (if in hospital). I personally do this every time as it makes me more involved in my own care. It's also really easy to forget what to ask when I don't have my list.

Alleviating dissatisfaction regarding your care or a treatment decision: If something doesn't sit right with you make sure you speak up quickly and directly and don't minimise it to yourself, or to the medicos. If you are not happy with a treatment decision or need more clarification about something, by all means discuss it further with the team. After further discussion, if you don't feel listened to or if your concerns aren't allayed you are well within your rights to seek a second (or third, or fourth) opinion. I have done just that regarding treatment for my pelvic complications and ended up seeking advice from four different colorectal surgeons. I chose not to have surgery at the end as there was no guaranteed fix.

Ultimately, YOU are the one who gets to have the last word regarding your care: It is well within your rights to say NO to a treatment decision, whether it involves medications, surgeries or other care options. In saying this, I would like to point out that medical professionals more often than not have your best interests at heart. I encourage you to make your decisions based on having received all the relevant information and when you feel that you completely understand the risks vs. benefits of refusing a treatment. After that, listen to your intuition and act accordingly.

The 'Take-Aways'

You are allowed to:
- feel scared and vulnerable
- be assertive

- ask questions
- seek independent medical advice
- ask for more time to decide on something major like surgery, if not life-threatening
- And ultimately, you are allowed to say NO!

PART SIX

REALLY GETTING TO KNOW
YOURSELF & YOUR CROHN'S

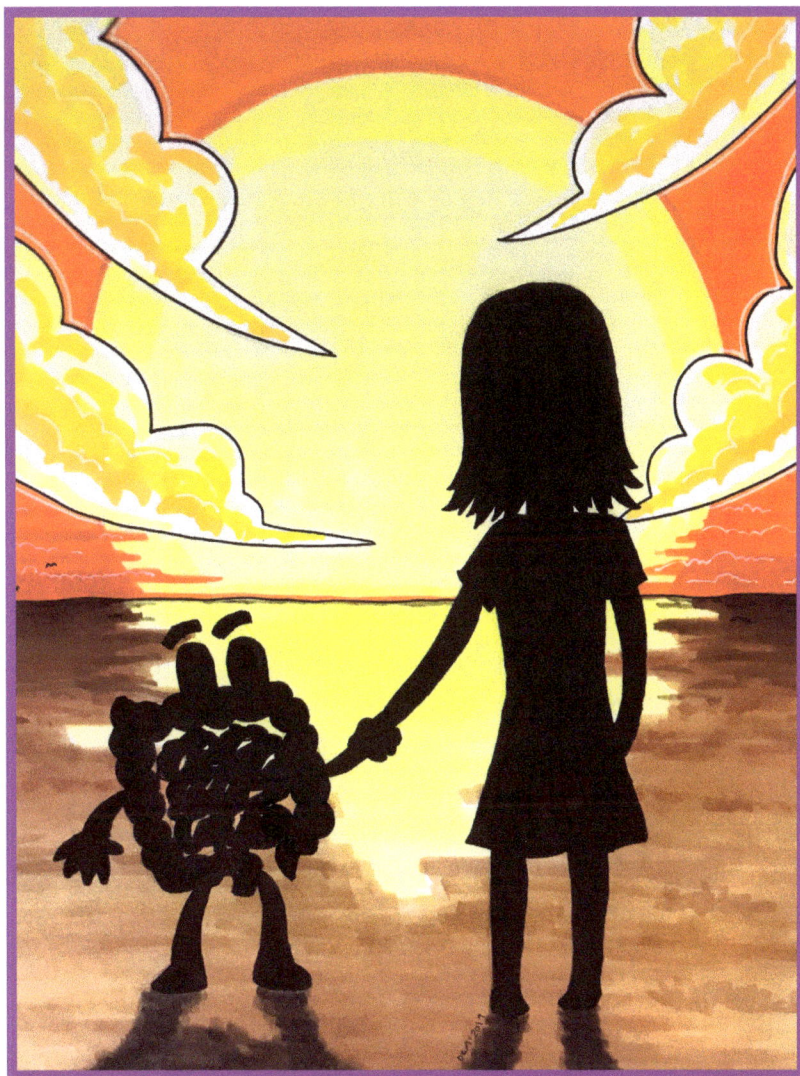

It really unsettles me that often we just "hand over our bodies" when we become a patient in hospital, whether it be due to an illness or when having a baby. By that I mean that a lot of us readily forfeit our involvement in our own health care and the associated decision making.

We don't speak up about how we feel or what we want because the medicos are experts after all and we trust that they will always know what's best for us. As a result, we can become completely disconnected from ourselves.

We stop listening to the messages our bodies are constantly sending us and ultimately, we stop 'hearing' them. We no longer follow our intuition; we don't assert ourselves or follow our instincts out of fear of being judged or labelled as 'difficult' by the medical world or because we have just become too passive with our own health. I really believe life would flow more effortlessly if we listened to our guts and asserted ourselves!

As both a long term Crohnie, AND a registered nurse, I have seen this phenomenon all too often. Just to paint a picture, I have come across so many patients in my 10 years of nursing who when asked what medications they were taking, would say something along the lines of "I don't know what medications I'm on, I just take whatever the doctor prescribes to me".

Why aren't we valuing ourselves and our health more?

Why aren't we learning about our conditions and how best to manage them?

The other thing that concerns me is that so many people don't really pay too much attention to their physical bodies or how they're feeling physically or mentally, until things grow bigger or the pain becomes too severe. In one way I think those of us with chronic illnesses like Crohn's disease are fortunate because over time we become so completely in tune with ourselves and we know our own bodies like the back of our hands so to speak.

To the newly diagnosed, I implore you to regularly check in with yourselves (mentally and physically), start to get to know your bodies, intimately, and proceed to forming a close, lifelong relationship with yourselves. I came across this quote a while back, I'm not sure who actually wrote it but it's so relevant and illustrates my point well,

"Listen to your body's whispers before they become screams."

Helpful Tips

Inspect your bodies regularly. I don't mean in a paranoid, "looking to find something bad" way, but in a loving way, in order to get to know yourself intimately. It's becomes easier to know when something is wrong, or out of balance, and it allows you to get on top of it quickly.

Work on accepting all of yourself! (hard, I know) You can't pick the bits you like and leave the rest. You come in a complete package – the 'good', the 'bad', and the 'ugly' so you might as well learn to love it all! Plus, our bodies do a lot for us every single day, so give thanks where thanks are due!

Check in with yourself and listen to your body first and foremost, then act accordingly! Find out what works for you (i.e. skin care, diet, etc.) so you can care for yourself the best you possibly can.

Learn your medications! Create a list of your medications (brand names and true names), their dosages and their frequency, along with what the medications are for, a simple explanation of what they do as well as their most common side effects. It's so important to understand what you are taking and also why, and when, to see your doctor.

Keep a health record: Let's face it, you have a chronic illness and it will become near impossible to remember all the bits and pieces regarding your treatment over the years. I keep a diary to record important dates (i.e. my diagnoses and previous surgery dates), my appointment outcomes, what dates I started taking particular medications (i.e. Humira or long courses of antibiotics), changes in my treatment plan, questions to ask at my next appointments, etc. This helped me out A LOT when I was really in the grips of my Crohn's, and spending so much time in hospital with flares, having my surgeries and other complications. I don't use it so much now.

As I mentioned previously, you know yourself the best out of everyone, so become your own advocate! No one else can do it better than you yourself can.

SO HERE WE ARE...

Phew! I honestly didn't think that I would finish this book, and at times (more often than not) I kept putting off writing because I was so overwhelmed by the sheer volume of information sitting in my head that was waiting to be regurgitated onto paper, and then into my computer.

Despite all my procrastination and self-doubt, I kept at it and I DID IT!!

And I am really proud of myself, as I believe very strongly in being able to pay forward my appreciation of the care and expert knowledge I have received from people along the way and to also pass on the knowledge I have acquired to others experiencing the grip of Crohn's right now.

It is 2019 as I write this and I am feeling well in myself, a huge part of this feeling comes from learning how to manage my health and anxiety attacks. I'm excited to say that my condition has stabilised (for now), so much so that my specialist has allowed me to stop taking my Crohn's medications. I have weaned off my anti-depressants, and my "second butt hole" has healed over—yah!

I mentioned near the start of the book that, at that time, I was planning a trip to Spain, well I did that, and while I was there I completed a 100 kilometre section of the El Camino trek as part of raising funds and awareness for Crohn's and Colitis Australia. I will not lie to you, it was bloody hard and like the writing of this book, there were days were I wanted to not get up and do it, but I am so happy I kept going on both of these adventures because they are two of the most rewarding things I have ever done.

So, to those of you struggling right now, you will get through it! I know at times it is incredibly difficult to believe but, just try to be as patient as you can be with the process and yourselves (whether it be during a flare up or recovery post-surgery), look after yourselves the best you can on your journey and try not to hold onto expectations of how you envision a certain outcome to be.

Things often work out, even if it's not how you initially imagined or hoped they would. At times I truly didn't think I would see the light at the end of the tunnel, but here I am!

Crohn's creates fighters!

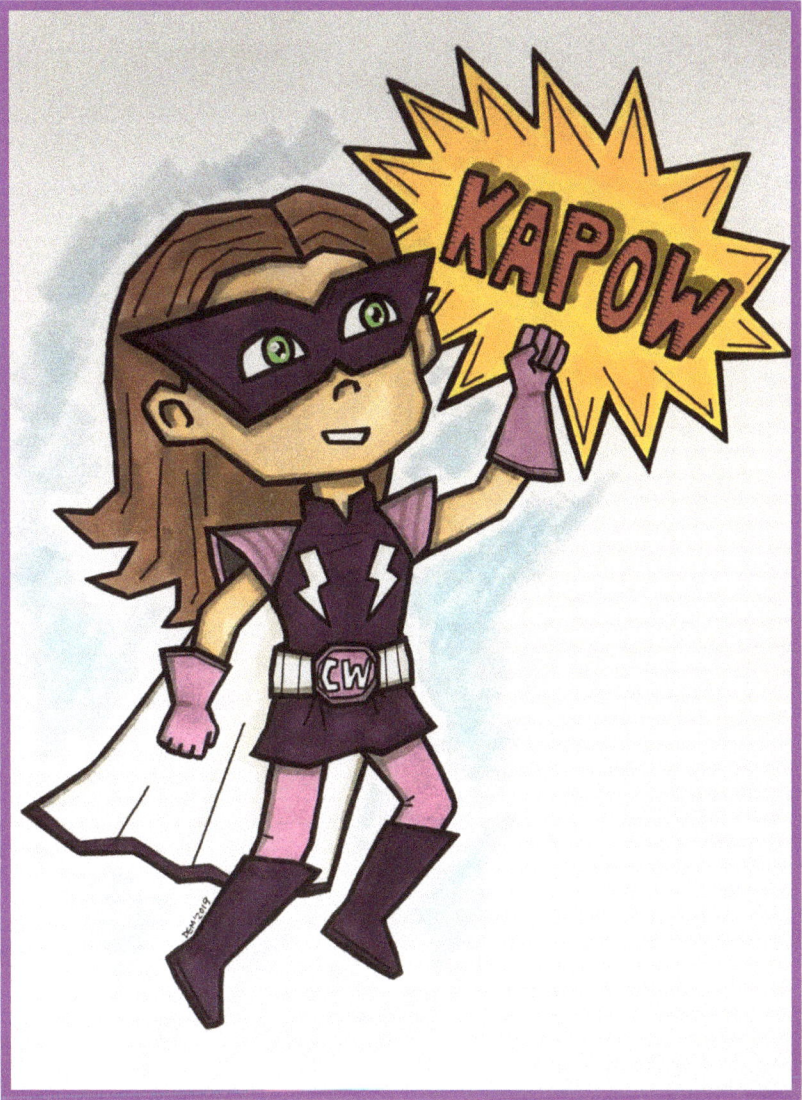

SHARING THEIR STORIES

In May 2018 I went to Spain to walk 113km on the El Camino over 5 days on behalf of Crohn's and Colitis Australia, accompanied by some very inspiring women who also have Crohn's disease.

They inspire me so much because they don't let their condition stop them from being positive, achieving their goals or from helping others. Connecting with these women certainly has helped me feel less alone because they know and understand what I go through day to day.

My advice is to surround yourself with people that inspire you, who don't allow their potential to be limited by their disease, who give you hope and motivate you to become the best version of yourself. Those who remind you that you are more than your diagnosis!

One of the things that really struck me about getting to know these ladies was the fact that we shared a lot of commonalities regarding our outlook on life and with the certain emotions, feelings, anxieties, annoyances and experiences we have each had in hospital and in daily life; but at the same time we are also vastly different in a lot of aspects regarding things such as: what area of the bowel our Crohn's has affected; our food intolerances; the type of surgeries we've had and the reasons why we had to have them; and the complications post-operatively or lack thereof; just to name a few.

To demonstrate how unique each person under the Crohn's umbrella really is, I have enlisted the help of one of the ladies –

Melissa, to share her story. Just like me, Melissa lives in Queensland, she has a permanent ileostomy; she is of a similar age and she is even looked after by the same specialists and stomal therapists as I, at the same hospital. She has kindly agreed to answer questions regarding her own Crohn's journey to help me highlight how unique each person's chronic illness experience is.

You'll see that yes, there are a lot of shared sentiments about certain things, but so many differences at the same time.

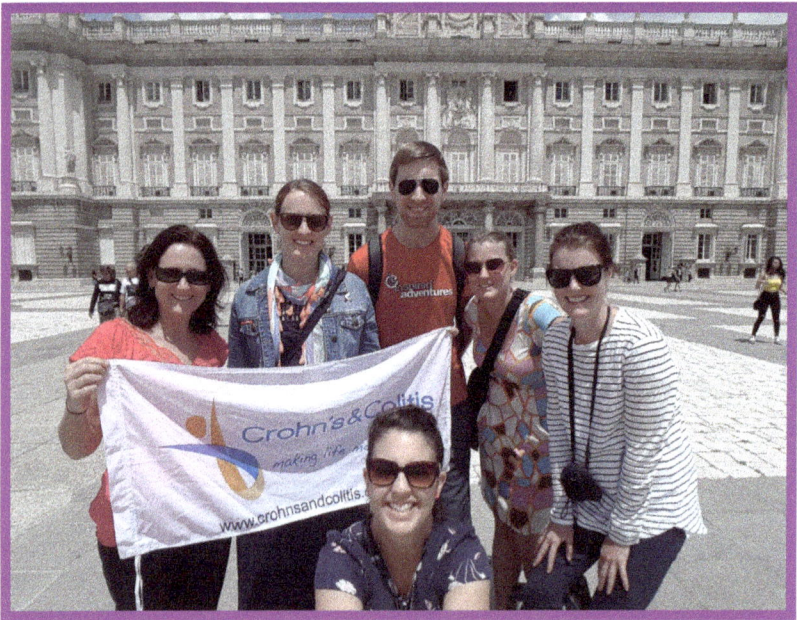

Taken in front of the Palacio Real in Madrid.
Clockwise from left: Desley (My mum), Lynsey, Jon, Me, Amy and crouching down is Melissa.

Melissa Lord (@gutlessandwonderful)
(Lockyer Valley, Queensland, Australia)

Q.1: Tell me about yourself and what you get up to?

A: I'm a mother of two boys who are aged 6 and 4. I've been married for eight years, but with my partner pretty much since high school. Family and friends are very important to me, so we spend a lot of time with our extended family and friends, even more so now we all have kids. So many birthday parties!

I work full time in communications for an elite sporting academy and it's an awesome workplace. Very supportive in regards to my health.

In the last 18mths I've started being a lot more active. I signed up for Parkrun, I registered to take part in a number of fun runs, including a 30km event last December. Being more active has led to us taking the kids on bushwalks and getting outdoors more, plus it's made me set goals - It's been great for me and my family.

Q.2: Where is your Crohn's and when were you diagnosed?

A: I'm currently in remission due to major surgery, however my Crohn's was located in my large bowel. I had some patches in my transverse colon with majority of instances in my descending and sigmoid colon, right down to my rectum and anal canal.

I was diagnosed in 2000, at the age of 18.

Q.3: Are you on regular medications?

A: Not presently. I haven't had any regular medications since having surgery.

Q.4: Other medical conditions?

A: I've had skin issues like dermatitis, anaemia, but no other significant conditions.

Q.5: Are there any foods that you can't tolerate?

A: Prior to surgery, most foods caused issues.

Post-surgery the foods that I can't tolerate include:

- ○ Chocolate – white chocolate is not so bad, but I still steer clear of chocolate as a rule. It causes my output to turn to water, I can also get mouth ulcers from it. Even the smallest piece has this affect.
- ○ Mango – can't digest it properly due to the fibrous texture and it causes blockages
- ○ Celery – similar to above, causes blockages
- ○ Field mushrooms – button mushrooms are okay, but I can't digest these properly and they cause blockages
- ○ Fresh tomato – I can eat Roma tomatoes, but normal tomatoes and cherry tomatoes or similar cause mouth ulcers due to their acidity. It does take a while to build up though, so I can eat some tomato without any affects but if I eat it every day, then I start having problems.
- ○ Anything super oily – makes my output more frequent
- ○ Garlic – I can tolerate it, but too much also causes frequent output and a lot of gas

Q.6: Do you suffer from any skin issues?

A: Growing up I suffered a lot from eczema and dermatitis. Not so much since surgery, I have the odd flare up, but nothing major.

Q.7: Do you swear by any products for skin issues?

A: These days I use QV 'soaps' and creams regularly. My son has a bit of dermatitis so I use them on him as well and find them great.

Q.8: Do you have a stoma?

A: Yes. I have a permanent ileostomy, surgery in November 2009.

Q.9: Are you happy with your stoma overall? Any problems?

A: Yes, I am. Best decision I ever made in the end. I was told at age 18 that I'd need this surgery and it was the worst thing anyone could have said to me. But I was uneducated about ostomy life at the time and a little naïve. I managed to avoid it for around 10 years thanks to some biological treatment, trial medications and steroids. However, there were a lot more bad memories from that time than good – in terms of my health.

My stoma has given me quality of life. I was healthy enough to fall pregnant and I had my boys. I can work full time, I can go to the shops without worrying about having an accident and best of all, my assumption that everyone would see/smell by bag was way off the mark – unless I tell people most are none the wiser. Not that I'm ashamed of it, I'll happily talk about it if I'm asked, but it just goes to show how little I knew back when I was first diagnosed. I have no regrets.

I've had a few issues over the years, including blockages and some skin irritation, but these are few and far between now as I've learnt what upsets me and I have my stoma care routine sorted. I've been using the same appliance (Coloplast Sensura Convex Midi, one piece) for years and I can trust it which is reassuring. Unless, of course, I self-sabotage by eating/drinking something I shouldn't.

Q.10: What Crohn's myth/s would you like busted?

A: The whole invisible disease element – the 'but you don't look sick' statement by those who have no clue about IBD.

Just because we may look 'well' on the outside bears no true reflection of the pain, anxiety and internal struggle of day-to-day life with Crohn's. Raising awareness, reducing stigma and changing perceptions is really important to me.

Conversations like these shouldn't be considered abnormal, there should be no taboo.

Q.11: Do you have a self-care routine (e.g.: exercise, diet, skin care)?

A: In the last couple of years exercise has definitely become part of my routine and I'm enjoying it. In terms of diet, it could be better, but to be honest I've been riding the wave of remission. I have a pretty good relationship with food these days and I love trying new things – a lot of which I couldn't do pre-surgery. Although I do have to be careful, I love a good cheese platter washed down with a wine!

Q.12: Anything that triggers your flare-ups?

A: I've had issues recently with giardia – as a result of our tank water. It's horrible and when I first had the bug I thought I was having a Crohn's flare and the alarm bells were ringing. I was so relieved when blood tests revealed it was a parasite.

I haven't had a flare since surgery. But beforehand stress was definitely a key trigger as well as food.

Q.13: As well as physically, does Crohn's affect you mentally, emotionally?

A: Yes. I don't mean to compare what I've experience to those who experienced severe trauma, but I do at times feel as though I've got a form of Post-Traumatic Stress Disorder. I'm quite anxious, a cautious worrier and often try and talk myself out of panic attacks. I have a habit of thinking the worst-case scenario, experience negative self-talk when in pressured situations and have low self-confidence, even if it doesn't come across that way. I put up a façade a lot – wear a mask that suits the situation.

I've had panic attacks after taking new medications because of the one instance I had anaphylaxis to Infliximab. Since then whenever I take anything new I panic that I'm going to have another severe reaction. Even if it's a different kind of paracetamol than I've had before.

Q.14: How do you stay positive?

A: Surround myself with my loved ones. My kids are always a great source of positivity, they make me proud and I want to make them proud.

Set goals and do my best to work towards them. Listen to music, it has a special way of pumping me up.

Also talking about my experiences has really helped in a way I didn't even know I needed. So I'm glad I started my Facebook and Instagram pages.

Q.15: Do you suffer from anxiety and depression?
A: I haven't been officially diagnosed, but yes, I think I do.

Q.16: How do you manage your mental health?
A: I've spoken over the phone to a psychologist before, but I've not sought regular help. However, it has become something I've thought more about doing recently.

Q.17: Do you have any advice for the newly diagnosed or in general?
A: Get educated. I was very uninformed about Crohn's and IBD and life as an ostomate. I kind of buried my head in the sand a bit and I wish I hadn't – so my advice is not to hide away from your diagnosis. Treatment and management of the disease has advanced so much.

Also, be your own advocate. Speak up for yourself and use your intuition. If something doesn't feel right then say so. Ask for a second opinion, it can't hurt.

Q.18: Any messages to the non-Crohn's population?
A: Be supportive, listen and stand by your loved one/friend who has been diagnosed.

In my experience I stayed at home a lot, and missed out on so many occasions, however my friends always stuck with me and didn't judge me. I'm so grateful for that and majority of them are still my best friends today. Some fall by the wayside, but true friends won't.

Understand that there is a difference between IBD and IBS. Crohn's and IBD are not IBS, nor can it be cured. It is a serious disease that has many knock-on effects, with medications and treatments that have almost as serious side effects. The cause is also not known and this is a major frustration for sufferers.

Crohn's sufferers still want to be active members of the society, however sometimes it's just not plausible. If someone admits their diagnosis to you, without sounding harsh, it's not an opportunity to tell that person ways to 'cure' their disease, or that someone you know used *insert alternative treatment here* to cure their Crohn's. It's just not that simple.

Q.19: Can you suggest any helpful resources or books that have helped you in the past?

A: There's no one specific resource unfortunately, I spoke to support groups, nurses, doctors and posted in online forums. I did find there was a lot more research and material to read from UK or American based sites – simply because they've been doing it for longer. Even the UK based Crohn's and Colitis organisation site is a good source.

I was lucky enough to have a visit from the Brisbane Ostomate Support Visitors Service prior to having surgery and it was amazing. I'd definitely recommend that.

Most recently, I've found the online IBD community to be amazing. I didn't really know how big it was until I created my Gutless and Wonderful accounts. Such a great resource, sure most of the people on there aren't doctors or nurses so can't give professional advice, but they can give you honest insight into life with this disease – hearing those real lived experiences are invaluable.

The more I think about it, us chronic illness warriors are the lucky ones. We were given these trials and challenges for a reason.

They have made us strong, they have made us resilient, they have made us wise, they have taught us to be grateful and appreciate our lives, they have made us become more in-tune with our bodies and seek out the best quality of life that we possibly can.

They have made us value and nurture ourselves.

They have given us depth.

I wouldn't change a thing.

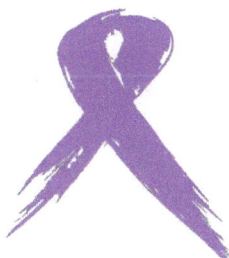

MEAGAN'S SURVIVAL SHOPPING LIST

Genital Psoriasis

Hope's Relief Premium eczema cream – moisturiser formulated for sensitive areas, fast absorbing and non-greasy. Apply a small amount once dry after showering.

Official website: https://www.hopesrelief.com.au/customer-service/faqs/

Lucas Paw Paw ointment – Creates a protective barrier and helps lock in moisturiser. Apply and spread along bottom crease.

Official website: http://www.lucaspapaw.com.au

Cavilon barrier wipes or spray – helps heal chronic splits and prevent further splitting. Apply, then dry with hairdryer to form protective film over split and surrounding skin.

Official website: https://www.3m.com.au

Cavilon No Sting Barrier Film is available free of charge on the Australian Stoma Appliance Scheme. Fill out the form on this page to request a sample: https://www.3m.com.au/3M/en_AU/cavilon-au/patients/ostomy/#Request_sample

Juju menstrual cup – during periods, helps keep my skin from sitting in menstrual blood for prolonged time.

Official site: https://www.juju.com.au

Sylk lubricant – natural ingredients. Helps protect my skin during sex and makes it more enjoyable.

Official site: http://www.sylk.co.nz

Psoriasis on knuckles

Doterra oils – 4 drops each of clary sage, lavender, frankincense, and tea tree oil into small container of Soft white paraffin. Apply to psoriasis areas just before bed.

Official Website: https://www.doterra.com/US/en

Peristomal Psoriasis

Welland Adhesive Remover Wipes – Tear open and add tap water to the mixture, then pour onto point where the bag and skin are glue to remove as much of the adhesive as possible before removing the bag. Once removed, I use the actual wipe to keep wiping the area the bag has been covering.

Online supplier: https://store.independenceaustralia.com/shop/Welland-Adhesive-Remover

Periorificial dermatitis

Soft white Paraffin – the only thing (paired with a clean wash cloth) I have found that I can tolerate on my face, especially when I have dermatitis flare ups. I use this as the base of a lot of my skin treatments.

Online supplier: https://www.amcal.com.au/david-craig-paraffin-soft-white---500g-p-9315676009303

Non-flare up facial routine

Moogoo Natural Skin Milk Udder Cream – daily after shower at night.

Official site: https://moogoo.com.au

French white clay – for exfoliating, once or twice a week, gently. https://www.healthandhappiness.com.au/online-shop/earthsgarden-diy-raw-ingredients/mineral-clay/australian-white-clay-kaolin-detail

Perianal Problems

Rectogesic ointment – Prescription only. Apply to anus. Relaxes the sphincter muscles and decreases the spasm and associated pain. Side effect: slight headache. Health Direct: https://www.healthdirect.gov.au/medicines/brand/amt,76016011000036108/rectogesic

Baby Wipes – for wiping up anal discharge, stronger than toilet paper, non-stick and they clean the area at the same time.

Official website: https://www.waterwipes.com/au/en/our-story-#online-retailers

Make up Pads - helps protect the perianal skin and soak up excess discharge. Fold in half and place in bottom crease.

Sitz (salt) baths - helps facilitate the drainage of muck from the bottom, helps manage infection and eases pain. Dissolve teaspoon of table salt in bath of warm water. Sitz bath definition: https://healthline.com/health/sitz-bath

Online supplier: https://www.wallcann.com.au/sitz-bath/

Pubic Pustules

pHisohex Anti-bacterial Wash – to kill bacteria in the infection. Wash area daily.

Official website: https://www.phisohex.com.au

Otocomb Otic Ointment – Prescription only. A combination of steroid medication and antibiotics. Apply sparingly to pustules after hot shower. Aspen Australia: https://www.ebs.tga.gov.au/

Bonus Bite!

Omnigon support garments range - Over the years, I have found that this range is ideal for multiple reasons including: hernia prevention (or to support a formed hernia) during exercise; concealing the stoma bag when you are wearing figure hugging clothing; and actually containing a stoma leak until you can get to a bathroom to clean yourself up (found this out one unfortunate day out). I personally use the moderate support waist bands under my work uniform; the moderate support briefs under my tighter "going out" clothes and jeans; and the moderate support boxers and the intermediate support briefs for when I go to the gym and yoga class. The garments are available free of charge on the Australian Stoma Appliance Scheme. Official website: http://www.omnigon.com.au/

REFERENCES

1. Crohn's disease definition (National Institute of Diabetes and Digestive and Kidney Diseases or NIDDK): https://www.niddk.nih.gov/health-information/digestive-diseases/crohns-disease

2. Functions of the skin (Ivy Rose Holistic): http://www.ivyroses.com/HumanBody/Skin/Functions-of-the-Skin.php

3. Psoriasis definition (Psoriasis Australia): http://www.psoriasisaustralia.org.au/about-psoriasis/

4. Link between Crohn's disease and psoriasis (National Psoriasis Foundation): https://www.psoriasis.org/advance/psoriasis-psoriatic-arthritis-connected-to-crohns

5. Genital psoriasis definition (DermNet NZ): https://www.dermnetnz.org/topics/genital-psoriasis

6. Periorificial dermatitis definition (DermNet NZ): https://www.dermnetnz.org/topics/periorificial-dermatitis/

7. Sugaring (Alexandria Professional): http://www.alexandriaprofessional.com/certification/wax-vs-sugar/

8. "The Inside Story: A toolkit for living well with IBD" (printed resource book) - Crohn's and Colitis Australia

9. Perforation definition (Medline Plus): https://medlineplus.gov/ency/article/000235.htm

10. Elevated liver enzymes definition (Mayo Clinic): https://www.mayoclinic.org/symptoms/elevated-liver-enzymes/basics/definition/sym-20050830

11. Myositis definition (Medline Plus): https://medlineplus.gov/myositis.html

12. Rhabdomyolysis definition (Health Direct): https://www.healthdirect.gov.au/rhabdomyolysis

13. Loop ileostomy definition (NHS): https://www.nhs.uk/conditions/ileostomy/

14. Neurologist definition (UR Medicine: Highland Hospital): https://www.urmc.rochester.edu/highland/departments-centers/neurology/what-is-a-neurologist.aspx

15. Endometriosis definition (BUPA Australia): https://www.bupa.com.au/health-and-wellness/health-information/az-health-information/endometriosis

16. Carrier of Duchenne Muscular Dystrophy definition (Duchenne Family Support Group): https://www.dfsg.org.uk/understand-dmd/manifesting-carriers-of-duchenne-muscular-dystrophy/

17. IVF definition (IVF Australia): https://www.ivf.com.au/fertility-treatment/ivf-treatment

18. Pan-proctocolectomy definition (Birmingham Bowel Clinic): http://www.birminghambowelclinic.co.uk/treatments-pan-proctocolectomy/

19. Sinus definition (The Free Dictionary): http://medical-dictionary.thefreedictionary.com/sinus

20. Lesser sciatic foramen definition (Radiopaedia): https://radiopaedia.org/articles/lesser-sciatic-foramen

21. Clear fluids definition (NSW Government: Agency for Clinical Innovation): https://www.aci.health.nsw.gov.au/__data/assets/pdf_file/0010/277039/diet-clear-fluids.pdf

22. Psyllium husk definition (Medical News Today): https://www.medicalnewstoday.com/articles/318707.php?sr

23. Wet wraps definition (DermNet NZ): https://www.dermnetnz.org/topics/wet-wraps/

24. Emollient definition (DermNet NZ): https://www.dermnetnz.org/topics/emollients-and-moisturisers/

25. Topical steroid cream definition (DermNet NZ): https://www.dermnetnz.org/topics/topical-steroid/

26. Erythroderma definition (DermNet NZ): https://www.dermnetnz.org/topics/erythroderma/

27. Anal spasm explanation (American Society of Colon and Rectal Surgeons): https://www.fascrs.org/patients/disease-condition/anal-fissure-expanded-information

28. Sitz bath definition (Healthline): https://healthline.com/health/sitz-bath

29. Pustule definition (Oxford dictionaries): https://www.oxforddictionaries.com

30. Folliculitis definition (DermNet NZ): https://www.dermnetnz.org/topics/folliculitis/

31. Sugaring definition (Oxford dictionaries): https://www.oxforddictionaries.com

Image Sources

1. Camino Trek 2018
https://www.crohnsandcolitis.com.au/how-to-help/fundraise/cca-el-camino-trek-2018/

2. Ileostomy diagram
https://www.dovemed.com/common-procedures/procedures-surgical/ileostomy/

3. Gut Issues
https://www.huffingtonpost.com/entry/the-gut-skin-axis-the-importance-of-gut-health-for_us_5983db63e4b00833d1de2703

4. Pelvic and Perianal issues
   https://www.practicalpainmanagement.com/patient/
   conditions/pelvic-pain/exams-test-diagnose-pelvic-pain

5. How to advocate for yourself
   https://www.lynda.com/Business-Business-Skills-tutorials/
   Learning-Assertive/175640-2.html

GLOSSARY

1   **Gastroenterologist:** "A doctor who specialises in the diagnosis and treatment of patients with gastrointestinal diseases" (CCA)

2   **Colorectal surgeon:** "A surgeon who specialises in diseases of the large intestine" (CCA)

3   **Stoma:** "A surgically-created opening whereby the intestine is brought out through the abdominal surface to allow drainage of intestinal contents" (CCA). Refers to a colostomy, ileostomy or urostomy.

4   **Stoma nurse/therapist:** "Nurses specially trained in the care of stomas" (CCA)

5   **Autoimmune disease:** "A condition characterised by an inflammatory reaction to one's own body tissue" (CCA)

6   **Ulceration:** "A break in the skin or in the lining of the gastrointestinal tract" (CCA)

7   **Stricture:** "A narrowed area of intestine usually caused by active inflammation or scar tissue" (CCA)

8   **Corticosteroids:** a class of medications that can be administered orally and intravenously and are most often used to control acute inflammation, for example during a Crohn's flare up. This includes prednisone and hydrocortisone.

9   **Immunomodulators:** "A group of medications that control inflammation by suppressing the immune system. Also known as immunosuppressives" (CCA). They are administered mostly orally, which includes Azathioprine (Imuran) and Mercaptopurine (6-MP or Puri-nethol).

10 **Biological Agents:** "A category of immunomodulator medications derived from living organisms and their products such as proteins, genes and antibodies that block the action of tumour necrosis factor-alpha (TNF-). Examples are infliximab (Remicade) and adalimumab (Humira)" (CCA)

11 **Perianal:** situated in or affecting the area around the anus.

12 **Fissure:** "A tear or break in a body surface; e.g. an anal fissure is a painful tear in the lining of the anus" (CCA)

13 **Fistula:** "An abnormal channel occurring between two loops of intestine, or between the intestine and another hollow structure such as the bladder, vagina or skin. Fistulae (plural) are more common in Crohn's disease than in ulcerative colitis" (CCA)

14 **Bowel perforation:** "Perforation is a hole that develops through the wall of a body organ. This problem may occur in the oesophagus, stomach, small intestine, large intestine, rectum, or gallbladder" (Medline plus)

15 **Terminal ileum:** "The lowest end of the small intestine before it joins the large intestine" (CCA)

16 **Colon:** "the large intestine or large bowel. The colon has five segments: caecum, ascending colon, transverse colon, descending colon and sigmoid colon" (CCA)

17 **Elevated liver enzymes:** "Elevated liver enzymes may indicate inflammation or damage to cells in the liver. Inflamed or injured liver cells leak higher than normal amounts of certain chemicals, including liver enzymes, into the bloodstream, which can result in elevated liver enzymes on blood tests" (Mayo Clinic)

18 **Balsalazide (Colazide):** part of a drug class known as Aminosalicylates, which are "a class of medications containing 5-ASA (5-aminosalicyclic acid) as the active component. Used to control inflammation in people with IBD" (CCA)

19 **Anal skin tags:** "Swollen lumps or 'flaps' of thickened skin that can occur just outside the anus in people with Crohn's disease" (CCA)

20 **Myositis:** "…inflammation of the muscles that you use to move your body. An injury, infection, or autoimmune disease can cause it. Two specific kinds are polymyositis and dermatomyositis. Polymyositis causes muscle weakness, usually in the muscles closest to the trunk of your body. Dermatomyositis causes muscle weakness, plus a skin rash" (Medline Plus)

21 **Rhabdomyolysis:** "…happens when muscle tissue is destroyed and the muscle fibres break down, releasing their contents into the bloodstream. This can lead to problems such as kidney failure. Rarely, rhabdomyolysis can cause death. However, when treated early, the chances of a recovery are high" (Health Direct)

22 **Temporary loop ileostomy:** "…where a loop of small intestine is pulled out through a cut (incision) in your abdomen, before being opened up and stitched to the skin to form a stoma" (NHS)

23 **Ileostomy/Stoma Bag:** "A surgical procedure whereby the ileum is brought out through an opening (stoma) created on the abdominal surface such that waste matter can drain into a bag fitted over the stoma" (CCA)

24 **Neurologist:** A doctor who "…treats disorders that affect the brain, spinal cord, and nerves" (UR Medicine: Highland Hospital)

25 **Endometriosis:** "The lining of a woman's uterus (womb) is called the endometrium. Each month the endometrium thickens under hormonal influence and then sheds during the monthly bleed (period). For reasons we don't yet understand, sometimes endometrial tissue grows outside the uterus—most commonly on the ovaries, fallopian tubes or inside the pelvis in an area between the uterus and the rectum. It may also grow on the bowel, bladder or elsewhere" (BUPA)

26 **Duchenne muscular dystrophy (carrier of):** "Although it is a commonly held belief that carriers merely pass on the disease and are unaffected, female carriers can have similar muscular weakness as affected males and for this reason are termed Manifesting

Carriers. This condition can occur with no known family history of DMD so all females who are suspected of having any form of muscular dystrophy should be tested to determine if they could be Manifesting Carriers because of the genetic implications" (Duchenne Family Support Group)

27 **IVF:** "… (In Vitro Fertilisation) is a procedure, used to overcome a range of fertility issues, by which an egg and sperm are joined together outside the body, in a specialised laboratory. The fertilised egg (*embryo*) is allowed to grow in a protected environment for some days before being transferred into the woman's uterus increasing the chance that a pregnancy will occur" (IVF Australia)

28 **Passing mucus from the rectum with a temporary ileostomy in place:** Despite the faecal matter being bypassed into a bag, if the large bowel or at least the rectum is still intact, it is still possible to pass mucus out of the bottom. Mucus is "a lubricant secreted by mucous membranes such as the inner lining of the intestine" (CCA). Mucus is constantly produced and it protects the intestinal wall from sustaining damage.

29 **MRI (magnetic resonance imaging):** "A type of non-invasive diagnostic technique that uses a strong magnet to produce computerised mages of internal body tissues" (CCA)

30 **CT/CAT scan (computerised axial tomography):** "A type of computerised x-ray machine that takes images from many different angles then assembles them to provide a three-dimensional image of internal structures" (CCA)

31 **Pan-proctocolectomy:** "This operation can be performed as an open or laparoscopic (keyhole procedure). During the operation the whole of the colon, rectum and anus are removed. This involves taking away the blood vessels and lymph nodes to that part of the bowel. As well as the abdominal incision patients will also have an incision around their bottom so that the surgeon can completely remove the anus" (Birmingham Bowel Clinic)

³² **Anal sphincters:** "A ring of muscle that surrounds an opening such as the anus". The anus contains both internal and external sphincters. (CCA)

³³ **Clear fluids:** "Only fluids or foods that liquefy at room temperature. All liquids containing fat are excluded…to replace or maintain the body's water balance and leave minimum residue in the intestinal tract" (NSW Government: Agency for Clinical Innovation). Patients who have had ileostomy surgery often commence a clear fluid diet post-operatively until their bowel is recovered enough to digest solid food again.

³⁴ **Sinus (surgical/perianal):** "An abnormal channel or fistula, permitting escape of pus" (The Free Dictionary). After my pan-proctocolectomy (where my large intestine, rectum and anus was removed), an open sinus/channel was left, which to this day still drains discharge.

³⁵ **CT guided Transgluteal drainage approach:** This procedure is performed on patients who have deep pelvic infections. It is guided by CT (thus avoiding nerves and blood vessels), where a drain is inserted through the gluteal muscle in the bottom, through a channel in the pelvis known as the sciatic foramen and into the pelvic cavity where the infection is sitting, in the attempt to drain the infected fluid.

³⁶ **(Lesser) Sciatic foramen:** "A small opening which provides communication between the pelvis and the gluteal region" (Radiopaedia)

³⁷ **Chia seeds:** an edible seed originating from regions in South America. High in fibre and omega-3 fatty acids. When soaked in liquid, the seed forms a mucilaginous coating with a gelatinous consistency.

³⁸ **Psyllium husk:** "Psyllium is a soluble fiber derived from the seeds of Plantago ovata, an herb mainly grown in India. It's used as a dietary supplement and is usually found in the form of husk, granules, capsules or powder" (Medical News Today)

39 **Pathogen:** "A micro-organism (bacterium or virus) capable of causing disease" (CCA)

40 **Dermatologist:** A doctor who specialises in the diagnosis and treatment of skin conditions.

41 **Wet wraps:** "'Wet wraps' are wet bandages wrapped over emollients and/or topical steroid creams to areas of red, hot, weeping eczema (most often due to atopic dermatitis). It may also be valuable in erythroderma, whatever its cause" (DermNet NZ)

42 **Anal spasm/pain (as a consequence of anal fissures):** "The typical symptoms of an anal fissure include **pain** and bleeding with bowel movements. Patients note severe pain during, and especially after a bowel movement, lasting from several minutes to a few hours" (American Society of Colon and Rectal Surgeons)

43 **Rectogesic ointment:** A prescription-only medication. The active ingredient in this ointment is glyceryl trinitrate (GTN), which acts on the blood vessels around the anus to relax them and prevent anal spasm.

44 **Sitz (salt) bath:** "A sitz bath is a warm, shallow bath that cleanses the perineum, which is the space between the rectum and the vulva or scrotum. A sitz bath can be used for everyday personal hygiene. It can also provide relief from pain or itching in the genital area" (Healthline)

45 **Pustule:** "a small blister or pimple on the skin containing pus" (Oxford Dictionaries)

46 **Folliculitis:** "...is the name given to a group of skin conditions in which there are inflamed hair follicles. The result is a tender red spot, often with a surface pustule. Folliculitis may be superficial or deep. It can affect anywhere there are hairs, including chest, back, buttocks, arms and legs. Acne and its variants are also types of folliculitis" (DermNet NZ)

47 **Sugaring:** "a method of removing unwanted hair by applying a mixture of lemon juice, sugar, and water to the skin and then peeling it off together with the hair" (Oxford Dictionaries)

www.ingramcontent.com/pod-product-compliance
Lightning Source LLC
Chambersburg PA
CBHW041300040426
42334CB00028BA/3093